Child Maltreatment Solutions Network

Series editor
Jennie G. Noll, Pennsylvania State University, University Park, Pennsylvania, USA

AF800468

More information about this series at http://www.springer.com/series/15457

Jennie G. Noll • Idan Shalev
Editors

The Biology of Early Life Stress

Understanding Child Maltreatment and Trauma

Springer

Editors
Jennie G. Noll
The Pennsylvania State University
USA

Idan Shalev
Department of Biobehavioral Health
The Pennsylvania State University
State College, PA, USA

ISSN 2509-7156 ISSN 2509-7164 (electronic)
Child Maltreatment Solutions Network
ISBN 978-3-030-10233-3 ISBN 978-3-319-72589-5 (eBook)
https://doi.org/10.1007/978-3-319-72589-5

© Springer International Publishing AG, part of Springer Nature 2018
Softcover re-print of the Hardcover 1st edition 2018
This work is subject to copyright. All rights are reserved by the Publisher, whether the whole or part of the material is concerned, specifically the rights of translation, reprinting, reuse of illustrations, recitation, broadcasting, reproduction on microfilms or in any other physical way, and transmission or information storage and retrieval, electronic adaptation, computer software, or by similar or dissimilar methodology now known or hereafter developed.
The use of general descriptive names, registered names, trademarks, service marks, etc. in this publication does not imply, even in the absence of a specific statement, that such names are exempt from the relevant protective laws and regulations and therefore free for general use.
The publisher, the authors and the editors are safe to assume that the advice and information in this book are believed to be true and accurate at the date of publication. Neither the publisher nor the authors or the editors give a warranty, express or implied, with respect to the material contained herein or for any errors or omissions that may have been made. The publisher remains neutral with regard to jurisdictional claims in published maps and institutional affiliations.

Printed on acid-free paper

This Springer imprint is published by the registered company Springer International Publishing AG part of Springer Nature.
The registered company address is: Gewerbestrasse 11, 6330 Cham, Switzerland

To Penelope K. Trickett, PhD, 1943–2016
and
Frank W. Putnam, MD
Mentors, colleagues and friends
who pioneered this work and changed many lives in doing so.

Acknowledgements

First, we would like to thank each one of the authors for their contributions: our sincere gratitude for your contribution and commitment to this book. Thank you for your willingness to share your time and expertise and for dedicating your careers to the betterment of children everywhere.

We would also like to thank the assistant director of the Child Maltreatment Solutions Network, Sandee Kyler, whose persistence and dedication made this book become a reality.

Many thanks go to the sponsors of the conference for their generous financial contributions including the Bennett Pierce Prevention Research Center; Clearinghouse for Military Family Readiness; Child Study Center; College of Information Sciences and Technology; College of Nursing; Department of Biobehavioral Health; Department of Education Psychology, Counseling, and Special Education; Department of Human Development and Family Studies; Penn State Public Health Sciences; and Pennsylvania Coalition Against Rape.

Finally, the unwavering love and support from Lydia Noll, Greta Noll, and Chad Shenk for keeping the stress at bay and the preciousness of life in focus (JN). To the vision, leadership, and support of Jennie Noll, Thomas Gould, and Nan Crouter from the College of Health and Human Development, Mrs. Edna Bennett Pierce for her combined vision and generous endowment, and last but not least, my beloved father, Moti Shalev, whom I miss dearly (IS).

The Pennsylvania State University
USA

Jennie G. Noll, Ph.D.
Idan Shalev, Ph.D.

Introduction to New Frontiers in the Biology of Stress

In Dostoyevsky's epic tale, Alyosha, the youngest and purest of Dostoyevsky's brothers Karamazov, is concerned that his brother Ivan has publically professed himself an atheist. With Alyosha being a monk, his brother's salvation is vitally important to him, and he implores Ivan to tell him why he has abandoned his faith. Ivan tells his brother that he simply cannot espouse belief in a benevolent creator who would knowingly allow children to suffer abuse. To make his case, Ivan goes on to describe graphic accounts of child abuse that he has witnessed throughout his travels. In the telling, Dostoyevsky doesn't stop at just two or three examples. He devotes pages and pages to five, six, seven chilling stories of children being victimized, with gruesome detail of unspeakable acts. One can't help wondering, "Why so many accounts? We got the point after the first five!" But Dostoyevsky is relentless, perhaps because he wanted to begin a conversation about child abuse in a way that is difficult to ignore or brush aside. Although published in 1880, the details of these accounts resonate even today. Yes, these stories are still all-too-familiar to those of you who work on the frontlines, those who do treatment, and those who seek to make sense of such stories. Rest assured, there are another 600 pages in which to decide if Ivan can rectify his faith crisis as Dostoyevsky presents redemptive examples of human decency and interventions on behalf of suffering children. He does this, perhaps, because he recognized that simply telling the story of an abused child does little good. It is what we *do* with the story that counts.

The same is true for knowledge. Knowledge does no good if it sits untranslated in academic journals or gets buried in jargon behind university walls. Likewise, knowledge does no good if it addresses unimportant questions or has little or no impact on a problem. Answering relevant questions that can generate workable solutions is, in fact, the chief responsibility of science. Translating these solutions into products that can be realistically implemented within the confines of the end-user environment is also of vital importance and is an all-too-often overlooked basic tenet of science.

The conference, titled "New Frontiers in the Biology of Stress, Maltreatment and Trauma: Opportunities for translation, resilience and reversibility," held on September 30—October 1, 2015, at Penn State's Nittany Lion Inn, brought together a group of scientists who are arguably the best researchers in the world on biological embedding. Also in attendance were some of the best in the world at translational messaging who will help transform this knowledge into workable, practical solutions for victims, practitioners, and future theorists. Finally, in attendance were brave, committed, and selfless individuals who have dedicated their lives to serving abused and neglected children on the front lines—social workers, child welfare workers, children and youth professionals, advocates, law enforcement, therapists, and pediatricians. We all came together to talk about the impact of abuse and neglect on our most vulnerable children, to discuss ways in which these lives—although profoundly affected by trauma and early life stress—can be set on a course of recovery, resilience, and hope. The commitment of all involved was to dedicate these few days, and our individual professional efforts, to the betterment of children. Until we can completely prevent child abuse and neglect from impacting the lives of children, those dedicated among us will work tirelessly to serve survivors using the best tools available to promote well-being and set in motion an optimal developmental course that holds the best promise for promoting healthy, productive lives.

There are the "stepping stones" of scientific impact—that is, taking ideas through the scientific method and then through implementation, refinement, and uptake. But we all know that this process can take years, even decades, before knowledge becomes useful. And in the meantime, more and more of Dostoyevsky's stories get told. This is why we brought basic scientists who work at the molecular level together with other scientists who understand the human processes of resilience and the possibilities for reversing the damage of stress, trauma, and maltreatment. This is why we so value the presence of practitioners, child welfare professionals, and advocates—to ensure that we are asking the right questions and working toward useful solutions. When we look at this problem through many different lenses, the science-to-practice process can be accelerated.

It might be helpful to imagine how, collectively, we might think of these as not merely "stepping stones," but rather "leaping stones." How, by coming together to have a conversation and produce a common language, we can help each other in accelerating the process of science and its translation. Like playing a game of leap-frog—where one person stoops on the ground and the other person leaps over, taking turns running and leaping over each other—by working together, the leaps made by a team can cover significantly more ground, more swiftly, than individuals would by leaping alone. In this way, we can think about our individual contributions to solutions and the ways in which we can facilitate change: when it is our turn to leap, and when we should be on the ground supporting the progress of others. Whether crafting a special issue of a journal, contributing to a data repository, or helping to recruit families for research, there are several examples of how we can help each other facilitate change for survivors and spark novel and sustained change. Collectively, we can make swift progress. Each of us plays an important role in solving complex problems in ways that will have a sustaining impact. On behalf of vulnerable and suffering children, we should be constantly reminded to keep the conversation going.

Although we may have the desire to help one another in greasing the skids of science-to-practice, we need to remember that we are all coming from different perspectives, and we serve different masters and have to satisfy different stakeholders. So we need to be patient, and we need to communicate effectively. In this way, we will maximize our collective success.

A few resources are specifically dedicated to keeping the cross-system conversation vibrant and productive. Assembling this distinguished team of authors for this volume is one such resource.

Novel research in the science of stress biology has opened exciting new avenues for understanding how stress "gets under the skin," providing real opportunities for translation. The fields of endocrinology/immunology, neuroscience, and genomics are, independently and together, advancing knowledge that will change the way we think about early life stressors, such as how child maltreatment and other forms of traumatic experiences become biologically embedded and can impact subsequent health, development, and well-being. This collective interdisciplinary science is grappling with the notion that there might be biologic explanations that characterize why some affected individuals are more susceptible than others to the deleterious impact of stress. More importantly, the fact that environmental buffers can explain some of these individual differences sheds light on the real possibility that early adversity can be interrupted, intervened upon, and even reversed. Understanding how *nurture* intersects with *nature* will spark critical innovation in how to curtail the acute impact of stress, maltreatment, and trauma, as well as how to prevent further deterioration.

The purpose of this volume is to showcase recent biological advancements related to child maltreatment and other forms of trauma and chronic stress. Three distinct sections will cover processes of biological embedding (i.e., endocrine system/immunology, brain development, and genomics). Emphasizing the endocrine system/immunology section, Jacinda Li and Andrea Danese focus on inflammation as a key mediating pathway on the development of psychopathology; Christine Heim discusses early life stress and the role of genetics and epigenetic changes in genes related to stress regulation; and Bruce Ellis provides an adaption-based approach to explain the mind's ability to adapt and problem-solve in stressful environments, which can enable some individuals to thrive under such stress. In the brain development section, Jacoba Rock, Charles Geier, Jennie Noll, and Michael De Bellis discuss a conceptual framework for understanding key neurobiological developmental effects in children who experience maltreatment and the role of PTSD in exacerbating the developmental impact of trauma; Ryan Herringa furthers the discussion of the effects of childhood maltreatment and PTSD on the brain's processing of threat; Olivia Altamirano, Alex Basile, and Victor G. Carriòn focus on pediatric PTSD with children who experience multiple stressors and novel interventions/treatments to successfully adapt to posttraumatic deficits. Within the genomics section, Andrèe-Anne Bouvette-Turcot, Michael J. Meaney, and Kieran J. O'Donnell review the data from both preclinical models and clinical studies of early adversity and epigenetic mechanisms.

A final section focuses on resilience from a multi-level, multidisciplinary perspective, including potential avenues for reversibility. Kan Long and George A. Bonanno provide a new conceptual framework for resilience that includes pre-adversity functioning, the actual aversive circumstances, post-adversity resilient outcomes, and predictors of resilient outcomes.

A final chapter details a panel discussion of the data and ideas presented in these four areas, in which discourse among panel and audience members was encouraged.

Translation is a fundamental, yet often elusive, principle of science. The content of this book strives to include an integrative "translation" and "future-directions" component with particular focus on (1) how this research can be understood in the context of serving and treating stress-exposed individuals, and (2) applicable strategies for prevention, mitigating injurious outcomes, and reversibility. With eclectic representation, this volume presents a unique opportunity to encourage a dialogue between expert researchers, trainees, and front-line practitioners—an essential process in illuminating the "next steps" in scientific inquiry and the evolution of scientific knowledge into real-world application and practice.

The Pennsylvania State University
USA

Jennie G. Noll

Contents

Contributors

About the Editors

Jennie G. Noll Ph.D., is a Professor in the Department of Human Development and Family Studies at Penn State University. She is also the director of the Penn State's Child Maltreatment Solutions Network and the Principal Investigator of the NICHD P50 Translational Center for Child Maltreatment Studies. Over the past 25 years, Dr. Noll has been the PI on NIH-funded research grants aimed at (1) the long-term developmental and physical health consequences of childhood sexual abuse, (2) pathways to teen pregnancy and motherhood for maltreated adolescents, (3) the cyber-hygiene and social media behaviors of abused teens, and (4) reversibility of neurocognitive deficits in abused and stress-exposed populations. Results from Dr. Noll's work have been used to inform public policy recommendations for child abuse prevention and treatment as well as research priorities put forth by the Institute of Medicine and policy statements by the World Health Organization. As its Director, Dr. Noll supports the strategic goals of the Child Maltreatment Solutions Network: to raise the rigor of science, change trajectories for victims, mobilize public investment in prevention and treatment, and train and inspire the next generation of scientists, practitioners, and advocates who will coalesce to solve the complex issue of child maltreatment.

Idan Shalev Ph.D., is the Mark T. Greenberg Early Career Professor for the Study of Children's Health and Development and an Assistant Professor in the Department of Biobehavioral Health at Penn State University and a faculty member with the Child Maltreatment Solutions Network at Penn State University. Dr. Shalev's research entails an interdisciplinary approach to identify mechanisms underpinning the biological embedding of stress across the lifespan. His research combines the disciplines of molecular genetics, endocrinology, neurobiology, and psychology. Specifically, his research tests the effects of stress from early life on change in telomere length and other biomarkers of aging across the life course, and the consequences of change in telomere system for physical and mental health problems. Dr.

Shalev's current work explores temporal differences in gene expression and epigenetic changes in response to environmental stressors in the lab, as moderated by early life stress. His research aims to inform new targets for intervention studies to reverse the damaging effects of stress on our body and mind. He is the author of more than 40 scientific articles and chapters and serves on the editorial board of *Telomere and Telomerase* journal.

About the Authors

Olivia Altamirano B.A., is an Assistant Clinical Research Coordinator for the Health and Wellness Study at Stanford University. Ms. Altamirano graduated in 2014 with a bachelor's degree in psychology, *summa cum laude* honors, from the University of California, Santa Cruz. She has been involved in work with children and minority communities for years. She has served as a tutor, teacher assistant, and mentor in urban and rural communities in California. Ms. Altamirano has experience working with low-income, first generation, English language learners and immigrant children and youth. She aspires to become a clinical psychologist who conducts research with, and is an advocate for, Latinos experiencing severe mental illness.

George A. Bonanno Ph.D., is a Professor of Clinical Psychology and Director of the Loss, Trauma, and Emotion Lab in the Department of Counseling and Clinical Psychology at Teachers College, Columbia University. Dr. Bonanno received his Ph.D. from Yale University in 1991. His research interests center on the question of how human beings cope with loss, trauma, and other forms of extreme adversity, with an emphasis on resilience and the salutary role of personality, positive emotion, and emotion regulatory processes. His research has been funded by the *National Institutes of Health* and the *National Science Foundation*. He co-edited the book, *Emotion: Current Issues and Future Directions* (Guilford), and recently authored *The Other Side of Sadness: What the New Science of Bereavement Can Tell Us about Life after Loss* (Basic Books).

Andrée-Anne Bouvette-Turcot Ph.D., is a postdoctoral fellow in the Department of Psychiatry at McGill University. She completed her Ph.D. (clinical and experimental psychology) at the University of Montreal. She is also a licensed clinical psychologist. Dr. Bouvette-Turcot's work focuses on child developmental trajectories and how they are influenced by environmental factors such as maternal history of early adversity, maternal well-being, socioeconomic status, and genotype. She is also interested in individual differences and seeks to identify which factors promote children's resilience and optimal development.

Victor G. Carrión M.D., is the John A. Turner, M.D. Professor and Vice Chair of Psychiatry and Behavioral Sciences at Stanford University and Director of the Stanford Early Life Stress and Pediatric Anxiety Program. He is on the faculty at both Stanford University School of Medicine and Lucile Packard Children's Hospital. His multidisciplinary research on the behavioral, academic, emotional, and biological late effects of experiencing trauma has led to the development and implementation of effective new interventions for treating children who experience traumatic stress. Using posttraumatic stress disorder (PTSD) as an anchor, Dr. Carrión is investigating, through longitudinal studies, the effects of stress on developmental physiology and brain development and function. He is a Co-Founder of the Center for Youth Wellness in San Francisco, where he served on the Board and chaired the Scientific Advisory Council. In 2011, he was appointed by California's Attorney General Kamala Harris to the Mental Health Oversight and Accountability Commission of the State of California, which he now chairs. He has received awards from the American Academy of Child and Adolescent Psychiatry, the American Foundation for Suicide Prevention, the National Association for Research in Schizophrenia and Affective Disorders, the National Institute of Mental Health, and the Silicon Valley Business Journal.

Andrea Danese M.D., Ph.D., is Head of the Stress and Development Lab and Senior Lecturer in Developmental Psychobiology and Psychiatry at the Institute of Psychiatry, Psychology and Neuroscience, King's College London. He is an investigator on the UK Environmental-Risk (E-Risk) Longitudinal Twin Study, which follows 2232 twins born in 1994–95, and on the Dunedin Multidisciplinary Health and Development Study, which follows 1037 individuals born in 1972–73. His research integrates epidemiological, neuroscience, and clinical methods to inform new interventions for individuals who experienced psychological trauma. Dr. Danese is also an active clinician and works as Consultant Child and Adolescent Psychiatrist at the National & Specialist CAMHS Trauma & Anxiety Clinic at the Maudsley Hospital, London, UK—a top-tier clinical service providing treatment to children with complex histories of trauma and trauma-related psychopathology.

Michael D. De Bellis M.D., Ph.D., is a Professor of Psychiatry and Behavioral Sciences with tenure in the Department of Psychiatry and Behavioral Sciences, Duke University Medical Center, and a licensed and board-certified child psychiatrist with specialty training in the neurobiology of child maltreatment and pediatric maltreatment-related posttraumatic stress disorder (PTSD). Additionally he studies the consequences of adolescent alcohol and substance use disorder on youth brain development. His specialties include pediatric brain imaging, PTSD, and depression, and neuroendocrinology. Dr. De Bellis has a continuing interest in the development of maltreated children and their risk for adolescent onset substance use disorders at Duke, where as a professor, he has led several federal grants related to these issues since 2003. He has published over 100 peer-reviewed papers on this work. His published seminal work, titled "Developmental Traumatology: Biological Stress Systems and Brain Development in Maltreated Children with PTSD," received the prestigious A.E. Bennett Award from the Society of Biological Psychiatry in 1998. He was the recipient of the 1999 Chaim Danieli Young Professional Award from the International Society of Traumatic Stress Studies for outstanding and fundamental contribution to the field of traumatic stress studies. He recently received the 2015 AACAP Child Maltreatment and Violence Committee Passion Award for Outstanding Commitment for Abused and Neglected Kids. He is a member of the American College of Neuropsychopharmacology, International Society for Traumatic Stress Studies, Society of Biological Psychiatry, and the American Academy of Child and Adolescent Psychiatry.

Bruce J. Ellis Ph.D., is Professor of Psychology and Anthropology at the University of Utah. As an overarching goal of his career, Dr. Ellis seeks to leverage knowledge from both evolutionary biology and developmental science to address core issues in developmental psychopathology, especially in relation to child and adolescent health. This work employs life history theory to model stress-health relations over the life course. A major emphasis of his research has been the development of Biological Sensitivity to Context theory and its recent extension the Adaptive Calibration Model, which focus on how our biobehavioral systems respond to specific features of family environments and the larger ecological context. Dr. Ellis' empirical work examines the impact of fathers, family relationships, and socioecological conditions on children's biological stress responses, timing of pubertal development, risky adolescent behavior and cognition, and related health outcomes. In addition to this basic research, he is interested in real-world applications in the form of theoretically based interventions.

Charles F. Geier Ph.D., is an Associate Professor of Human Development and Family Studies and Neuroscience at Penn State University, and currently holds the Dr. Francis Keesler Graham Early Career Professorship in Developmental Neuroscience. His research examines neurodevelopmental changes in the interaction between cognitive and affective brain systems, and how this relates to decision making and risky behavior in adolescents and young adults.

Christine Heim Ph.D., is Professor and Director of the Institute of Medical Psychology at Charité Universitätsmedizin Berlin. Dr. Heim is also a Member of the Cluster of Excellence "Neurocure" at Charité in Berlin as well as Professor of Biobehavioral Health and Member of the Network on Child Protection and Well-being at Penn State University. Her research is focused on the neurobiological consequences of early-life trauma and their relationship to the development of depression, anxiety, and functional somatic disorders. The impact of her work is acknowledged in more than 14,000 citations. She is the recipient of several honors and awards, including the 2015 Patricia Barchas Award in Sociophysiology of the American Psychosomatic Society. She is an elected member of the American College of Neuropsychopharmacology. She is the recipient of multiple federal grants and foundation grants, and she serves on numerous national and international scientific review committees regarding research on the consequences of childhood trauma.

Ryan Herringa M.D., Ph.D., is an Assistant Professor in the Department of Psychiatry at the University of Wisconsin School of Medicine and Public Health. He is a pediatric psychiatrist and neuroscientist whose work explores the neural substrates of childhood traumatic stress and PTSD. He directs the BRAVE Youth Lab (Building Resilience after Adversity in Youth), which seeks to map neurodevelopmental trajectories following childhood trauma. Specifically, the BRAVE Lab uses structural and functional neuroimaging combined with behavioral, physiological, and genetic approaches to develop biomarkers of vulnerability, recovery, and resilience to childhood trauma. Biomarkers of childhood trauma could then be used to improve prevention and intervention strategies in victimized youth. In addition to his research, Dr. Herringa remains active in clinical care and teaching, with specialization in the treatment of youth with trauma-related mental illness.

Jacinda C. Li M.S., is a doctoral student in Human Development and Family Studies at the Pennsylvania State University. She works with Dr. Jennie Noll to study the bio-psycho-social consequences of childhood sexual abuse across the lifespan. Jacinda's research interests center on mechanisms that may underlie the development of various adverse health outcomes in female survivors of childhood sexual abuse with an emphasis on stress physiology and obesity.

Kan Long M.A., is a clinical psychology doctoral student in the Department of Counseling and Clinical Psychology at Teachers College, Columbia University.

Michael J. Meaney Ph.D., is a James McGill Professor of Medicine at Douglas Mental Health University Institute of McGill University. Dr. Meaney is the Director of the Maternal Adversity, Vulnerability and Neurodevelopment Project and of the Developmental Neuroendocrinology Laboratory of McGill University. He also joined the Singapore Institute for Clinical Sciences in 2008 as a Senior Investigator and leads the Integrative Neuroscience Program. Dr. Meaney's primary research interest is that of the stable effects of early experience on gene expression and development, focusing on the influence of variations in maternal care. These studies have led to the discovery of novel epigenetic mechanisms for the influence of early experience. His research is multidisciplinary and includes studies of behavior and physiology, to molecular biology and genetics. In 2012, Meaney was awarded the Order of Canada, the nation's highest citizen honor and the Distinguished Scientist award from the American Psychological Association. He currently holds a CIHR Senior Scientist Award. More recently, in 2014, he was awarded with the Klaus J. Jacobs Research Prize, the Prix Wilder-Penfield, and the Lifetime Achievement Award from the International Society of Psychoneuroendocrinology (ISPNE). The Meaney lab was designated as a "Mostly Highly Cited Researcher" in neuroscience by the Institute for Scientific Information. Graduates from Meaney's lab hold faculty appointments across North America, Asia, and Europe, including Columbia University, Queen's University, University of California at Berkley, University of British Columbia, University of Michigan, University of Pennsylvania, University of Toronto, INSERM (France), and the RIKEN Institute of Japan.

Kieran J. O'Donnell Ph.D., is an Assistant Professor in Epigenetics and Epidemiology within the Department of Psychiatry at McGill University (Canada). O'Donnell is a Canadian Institute for Advanced Research Global Scholar in Child and Brain Development and a Principal Investigator in the Ludmer Centre for Neuroinformatics and Mental Health. O'Donnell's group seek to better understand how early experience shapes vulnerability for later adverse mental health outcomes. Specific areas of interest include maternal perinatal mental health and child emotional/behavioral development, as well as incorporating molecular analyses within programs of early intervention with established clinical efficacy. The goal is to integrate informative biological measures into studies of child development to help each child reach their full developmental potential.

Jacoba Rock L.C.S.W., is a doctoral student of Human Development and Family Studies at Pennsylvania State University. She studies adolescent development, psychosocial and biological contributions to the development of offending behaviors, and opportunities for intervention with aggressive juveniles and young adults. Jacoba has a special interest in the empirical relationship between childhood trauma and violence in adolescence and adulthood. As a social worker in the state of Colorado, Jacoba worked with juveniles accused or convicted of violent crime, and advocated for their reverse transfer or re-sentencing, as well as access to mental health services and family contact, infusing sociological and developmental research into the courtroom and other decision-making systems. Jacoba also taught graduate Social Work and Criminology, supervised other social workers, and volunteered as a restorative justice facilitator for high-risk dialogue between victims and offenders.

Chapter 1
Biological Embedding of Child Maltreatment Through Inflammation

Jacinda C. Li and Andrea Danese

1.1 Introduction

The effects of trauma, maltreatment, and early-life stress on the immune system have gained increasing attention in research and clinical settings (Danese & Baldwin, 2017; Danese & Lewis, 2017). Exploring the effects of early-life stress on the immune system may uncover new targets for prevention and treatment of childhood traumatic stress-related psychopathology.

This chapter will provide a broad introduction to early-life stress and the immune system. First, the chapter will provide an overview on the relation between early-life stress and immunology. Next, relevant biological studies will be briefly summarized. Finally, the clinical implications of these biological studies will be discussed.

This chapter will illustrate the effects of early-life stress on the immune system as possible mediating pathways for the relation between childhood maltreatment and depression. Although a substantial amount of evidence exists to show that maltreatment is one of the key risk factors for the development of depression later in life (Widom, DuMont, & Czaja, 2007), specifically *how* maltreatment might contribute

J. C. Li
Department of Human Development and Family Studies, The Pennsylvania State University, University Park, Pennsylvania, USA
e-mail: jcl270@psu.edu

A. Danese (✉)
Social, Genetic, and Developmental Psychiatry Centre, Institute of Psychiatry, Psychology, and Neuroscience, King's College London, London, UK

Department of Child and Adolescent Psychiatry, Institute of Psychiatry, Psychology and Neuroscience, King's College London, London, UK

National and Specialist CAMHS Trauma and Anxiety Clinic, South London and Maudsley NHS Foundation Trust, London, UK
e-mail: Andrea.Danese@kcl.ac.uk

© Springer International Publishing AG, part of Springer Nature 2018

J. G. Noll, I. Shalev (eds.), *The Biology of Early Life Stress*, Child Maltreatment Solutions Network, https://doi.org/10.1007/978-3-319-72589-5_1

to the risk for depression is still unclear. This chapter will suggest that the immune system, particularly inflammation, may be one of the key mediating pathways that might explain the effects of childhood maltreatment on depression.

1.2 What Is Inflammation?

Innate immunity is an evolutionarily well-conserved component of the immune system. It has been shaped by the natural selection process because of repeated encounters of humans and their ancestors with common environmental pathogens throughout evolution. As a result of these encounters, innate immunity provides protection against common environmental pathogens to humans from their time of birth.

The innate immune system comprises a number of different elements. The *body physical barriers*, which include the skin and the gastrointestinal tract, separate the internal body environment from the external environment. The *non-self recognition elements*, which include the complement system and the toll-like receptors, recognize foreign entities that enter the body and then trigger the activation elements. The *activation elements*, which include the cytokines and the endothelial and other cells, contribute to the activation of the inflammatory response. This inflammatory response in turn triggers the response elements. The *response elements*, which include the phagocytes and the acute phase proteins, drive the innate immune response against the invading pathogens.

In cases of physical wounds and traumas, inflammation constitutes a vital response for preventing the spread of infection and for promoting tissue repair. The activation of the inflammatory response leads the liver to secrete several acute phase proteins, such as the response elements C-reactive protein (CRP) and fibrinogen. These response elements are released into the circulatory system and travel to the location of the wounds to combat infections. These response elements can also be relatively easily measured in the blood. As the end-products of the cascade of immune response events, the response elements can be measured to obtain information about the degree of activation of the inflammatory response.

1.3 Inflammation and Depression

How is inflammation related to the development of psychopathology? Consider the pathophysiology of depression, for example. Several molecular theories exist for explaining the processes by which inflammation may lead to depression. Figure 1.1 depicts one of the top theories developed over the last several years based on research in animal and humans models (Dantzer, O'Connor, Freund, Johnson, & Kelley, 2008; Miller, Maletic, & Raison, 2009). This theory centers on the role of the amino acid tryptophan. Tryptophan is the key precursor for the synthesis of serotonin, a neurotransmitter crucially involved in mood regulation. The significance of serotonin in mood regulation is, for example, supported by the clinical efficacy of the selective serotonin reuptake inhibitors (SSRIs), which increase the

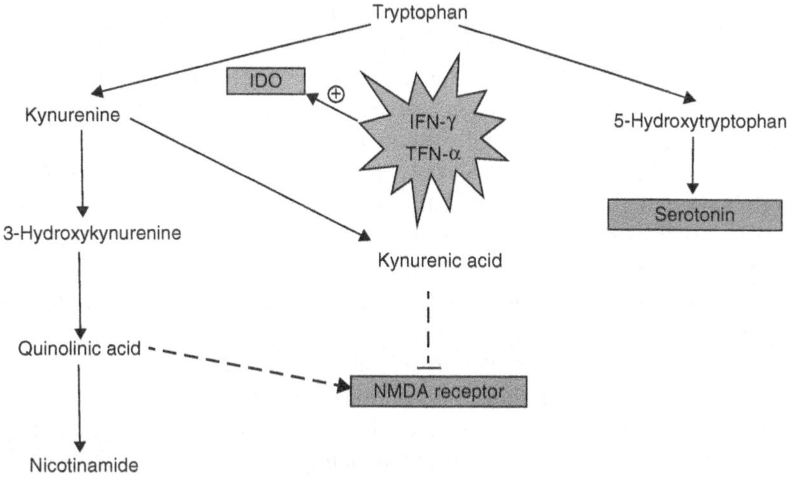

Fig. 1.1 Molecular theory of the effect of inflammation on depression through tryptophan. *IDO* indoleamine 2,3-dioxygenase, *IFN-γ* interferon (IFN)-γ, *TNF-α* tumor necrosis factor-α, *NMDA receptor* N-methyl-D-aspartate receptor. Figure adapted from Dantzer, R., et al. (2008). *Nature Reviews Neuroscience, 9*, 46–56

levels of serotonin in the synapse by inhibiting its reuptake through the serotonin transporter. In conditions of systemic inflammation, serum levels of the pro-inflammatory cytokines (i.e., response elements) interferon (IFN)-γ and tumor necrosis factor (TNF)-α are elevated. These cytokines stimulate an enzyme called indoleamine 2,3-dioxygenase (IDO). The IDO enzyme shunts tryptophan away from the synthesis of serotonin into an alternative path involving the synthesis of kynurenine. This path eventually leads to the stimulation of the N-methyl-D-aspartate (NMDA) receptor. The overstimulation of the NMDA receptor leads to its excitotoxicity, a pathological process that leads to neuron damage and deaths (Miller et al., 2009). Neuronal damage, including atrophy and loss of neurons and glia in the brain, is a key feature of the pathophysiology of depression (Miller et al., 2009). Therefore, conditions of systemic inflammation may bring about depression by lowering levels of serotonin and increasing the stimulation of the NMDA receptors. Other mechanisms also likely exist that contribute to the effect of inflammation on depression, as well as on a range of other psychiatric conditions. A comprehensive review of existing mechanisms, however, is beyond the scope of this chapter.

1.3.1 Studies in Humans on the Relation Between Inflammation and Depression

Given that inflammation might play an important role in the pathophysiology of depression, it can be expected that individuals in a clinical setting (i.e., patients) with depression would display higher levels of inflammation compared to patients without depression or nondepressed control individuals in a community setting.

Howren, Lamkin, and Suls (2009) conducted one of the existing meta-analyses that investigated the associations between depression and several key biomarkers of inflammation in community and clinical samples. The meta-analysis found that, compared to nondepressed adults, depressed adults displayed a statistically significant elevation in plasma levels of the following biomarkers: CRP (Cohen's $d = 0.15$, 95% confidence interval [CI]: 0.10–0.21, $p < 0.001$), interleukin (IL)-6 ($d = 0.25$, 95% CI: 0.18–0.31, $p < 0.001$), IL-1 ($d = 0.35$, 95% CI: 0.03–0.67, $p = 0.03$), and IL-1ra ($d = 0.25$, 95% CI: 0.04–0.46, $p = 0.02$). Because these data were correlational, however, the causal direction of these associations—inflammation leading to depression or depression leading to inflammation, or the existence of a bidirectional influence—could not be clarified.

Thus, experimental studies in both animal models and humans are essential for clarifying the direction of these associations. One such experimental study in humans was conducted by Musselman et al. (2001). This study was one of the first to show that the clinical use of pro-inflammatory cytokines for treating different types of cancer might induce depression in adults. In this double-blind study, 40 patients with diagnoses for malignant melanoma but no depression at the beginning of the study underwent therapy with cytokine interferon alfa, which stimulates the body's immune system. These patients were randomly assigned to receive either a placebo or the SSRI antidepressant paroxetine. After the first 12 weeks of the interferon-alfa therapy, the researchers observed among the cancer patients with no prior history of depression a progressive increase in the risks for major depression, as indicated by the reduction over time in the proportion of the sample that was free of diagnoses of major depression. This decline in the proportion of those free of depression was particularly pronounced among the patients who had received the placebo. The group that received the SSRI paroxetine, however, maintained a higher proportion of patients who were free of major depression, indicating that the administration of paroxetine may have partially buffered the effect of interferon-alfa therapy on risks of depressive symptoms. These findings suggest that compensating for some of the biological pathways through which inflammation may lead to depression (i.e., compensating for the reduced synthesis of serotonin with inhibited reuptake from the synaptic cleft) might help to reduce inflammation-induced risks of depression.

1.4 Child Maltreatment and Inflammation

In the effort to investigate the potential mediating role of inflammation in the association between childhood maltreatment and depression, it is important to test whether childhood maltreatment is associated with later inflammation. Similar to physical infections and tissue damage, acute and chronic psychosocial stress akin to maltreatment can trigger the inflammatory response. Exposure to stress triggers the activation of the sympathetic nervous system. The sympathetic nervous system, a component of the peripheral nervous system, leads to the activation of the inflammatory response. Stress-induced activation of the inflammatory response is considered an evolutionarily conserved mechanism through which exposure to psychosocial stress prepares the body to face tissue damage and infections, should they occur. In the modern day, however, perceptions of stress are not often accompanied by physical injury. Thus, the ability to "switch off" the inflammatory response becomes critical to maintaining homeostasis because inflammation, while a powerful tool to destroy foreign particles from the environment, is also a nonspecific response that can attack one's own body. Chronic exposure to inflammation may eventually contribute to cardiovascular disease, diabetes, and potentially dementia (Danese & McEwen, 2012). The body has redundant pathways aimed at inhibiting inflammation. One pathway is the activation of the parasympathetic nervous system (PSNS), a different branch of the peripheral nervous system. The other pathway is the activation of the hypothalamic-pituitary-adrenal (HPA) axis, which results in the secretion of the glucocorticoid cortisol. Cortisol is one of the most powerful anti-inflammatory compounds in the body. It is also used pharmaceutically to treat inflammatory conditions. The effectiveness of cortisol in fighting inflammation is very important in the context of maltreatment because adults with a history of childhood maltreatment also have impairment in the function of the HPA axis, potentially due to the relative resistance of the glucocorticoid receptor to the effect of cortisol (Heim, Newport, Mletzko, Miller, & Nemeroff, 2008). The resistance of the glucocorticoid receptor to cortisol may mean that even if the levels of the hormone cortisol were normal, or perhaps even elevated, in adults with a history of childhood maltreatment, these elevated levels of the hormone do not translate into increased effects of the hormone. It is then possible that adults with a history of childhood maltreatment may also have high levels of inflammation due to the impaired functioning of this anti-inflammatory pathway involving the HPA axis.

1.4.1 Epidemiological Studies for Child Maltreatment and Inflammation

This section will describe two studies in humans that examined the association between exposure to childhood maltreatment and risks for inflammation in adulthood.

Danese, Pariante, Caspi, Taylor, and Poulton (2007) investigated the life-course association between childhood maltreatment and adult inflammation in a birth cohort as part of the Dunedin Multidisciplinary Health and Development Study. The Dunedin Study is life-course study that began in Dunedin, New Zealand in 1972–1973 with a representative birth cohort of a thousand participants who were followed over their life course. The outcome measures for inflammation were drawn from participants when they were 32 years of age and included clinically relevant biomarkers of inflammation, such as high sensitive C-reactive protein (hsCRP), fibrinogen, and white blood cell counts (WBC). These indicators of inflammation are commonly used by physicians to predict the risks of developing cardiovascular diseases. The prospective longitudinal study design allowed for the number of childhood maltreatment experiences to be prospectively measured.

The childhood maltreatment indicator was a composite score of experiences that occurred between the ages of 3 and 11. Maternal rejection was measured by a clinical psychologist who observed the relationship between the mothers and the children starting when the children were age 3. Harsh discipline was measured using the parenting questionnaires when children were ages 5 and 7. Out of the sample-wide distribution, the top decile was calculated to identify the parents who, for that context and time, were particularly harsh to their children. Disruptive caregiver changes refer to repeated changes in primary caregivers, mainly caused by child protection concerns. Reports of physical and sexual abuse were obtained retrospectively from study participants at age 26 years. Although retrospective in nature, these reports of abuse were obtained prior to the outcomes of inflammation biomarkers and thus were unlikely to bias the results of the analyses. The cumulative prevalence of the abuse indicator revealed that three out of ten study participants experienced one of these childhood maltreatment experiences, and one of ten study members experienced two or more. Analyses were conducted based on the categories of no, probable, or definite maltreatment.

The first aim of the study was to examine the association between maltreatment and high levels of hsCRP (defined as greater than three milligrams per liter), which is a key risk factor for later cardiovascular disease. This definition for a high level of hsCRP has been endorsed by the Centers for Disease Control (CDC) and the American Heart Association as a reliable screening measure for risks of cardiovascular disease (Pearson et al., 2003). The results of these analyses showed that exposure to maltreatment was associated with a greater risk of high levels of hsCRP in adulthood. Participants who were classified in the category of individuals who had "probable" childhood maltreatment exposure had only a slightly increased, but not statistically significant, risk of having high levels of hsCRP (21.3% of the group had high hsCRP levels) compared to participants who had no childhood maltreatment exposures (18% of the group had high hsCRP levels). However, participants who were classified in the category of individuals who had "definite" childhood maltreatment exposures (i.e., a more extreme form of maltreatment), had a significantly greater risk of having high levels of hsCRP (32.5% of the group), and were almost twice as likely to have high levels of CRP in adulthood when compared to participants who had no childhood maltreatment exposure [risk ratio (RR) 1.80, 95% confidence interval (CI) 1.26–2.58].

Given that these results were based on long-term associations that might have included numerous intervening events between childhood and adulthood, alternative hypotheses to explain the association between childhood maltreatment and inflammation in adulthood were also tested. A common hypothesis from the literature is that maltreated children experience a cluster of early-life risk factors (Widom, 1989), including low birth weight (Sattar et al., 2004), socioeconomic disadvantage (Taylor, Lehman, Kiefe, & Seeman, 2006), and low intelligence quotients (IQ) (Whalley & Deary, 2001), which are independently associated with inflammation later in life. It is then possible that, rather than maltreatment having an effect on inflammation later on in life, other factors that were correlated with both maltreatment and inflammation could have explained the association observed. Furthermore, maltreated children are more likely to experience stress (Kiecolt-Glaser et al., 2003) and depression (Ford & Erlinger, 2004) in adulthood and to live in disadvantaged socioeconomic conditions (Steptoe, Owen, Kunz-Ebrecht, & Mohamed-Ali, 2002). Because these conditions occur in adulthood rather than childhood, they are not an alternative explanation (confounding). Rather, they highlight the potential processes by which maltreated children might develop high levels of inflammation (mediation). Depression and perceived stress are both also independent predictors of inflammation. Finally, maltreated children are more likely to have poor general health and health behaviors. For example, maltreated children are more likely to develop metabolic syndrome and smoke as adults. Some of these factors, again, independently predict inflammation. Of note, even after accounting for all of the above alternative hypotheses in regression analyses, the association between childhood maltreatment and a high level of CRP remained significant.

Still, questions remain regarding whether the association between childhood maltreatment and inflammation relies on only one measure of inflammation or can be generalized to other measures of inflammation. Thus, continuous measures of inflammation were then examined as outcomes to indicate not only *whether* high levels of inflammation exist but also *how much* inflammation exists. Thus, the test of the association between childhood maltreatment and inflammation was extended to continuous measures of hsCRP, fibrinogen, and WBC. Results showed that the significant association between childhood maltreatment and inflammation could be generalized to the continuous measures of hsCRP, fibrinogen, and WBC, suggesting that the association between childhood maltreatment and inflammation was not sensitive to a particular measure. Finally, the variances of all three biomarkers were combined into one factor calculated using principle component analysis, with the assumption that what was shared between three biomarkers of inflammation more specifically measures inflammation. Even with this more specific measure of inflammation, significant and graded associations between maltreatment and inflammation remained. In summary, these analyses indicated that childhood maltreatment might help to identify individuals in the population who have high levels of inflammation.

In order to test the research question regarding whether childhood maltreatment could contribute to identifying subgroups of individuals with depression who also have elevated inflammation levels, Danese et al. (2008) again utilized the Dunedin Study data. The following groups of individuals were examined: (1) those who did not have a history of maltreatment or depression to serve as controls; (2) those who had only depression, but no maltreatment; (3) those who had maltreatment but no depression; and (4) those who had both maltreatment and depression. The researchers tested the association between those being classified in each of these groups and having a high inflammation level as indexed by a level of hsCRP greater than three milligram per liter. In the sample, high levels of hsCRP were found in 17.9% of the control group, 25% of participants who had only depression, 30.4% of participants who had only maltreatment, and 37% of participants who had depression and maltreatment. Among the four groups of participants, those who only had depression had a small, not statistically significant, increase in the risk of having high hsCRP levels (relative risk [RR] 1.40; 95% CI: 0.97–2.01). However, those with maltreatment only (RR 1.45; 95% CI: 1.06–1.99), and to an even greater extent those with maltreatment and depression (RR 2.07; 95% CI: 1.23–3.47), had significantly elevated risks of having high hsCRP levels. These findings suggest that maltreatment may not only be useful for identifying individuals with high levels of inflammation in the general population, but may also have similar potential in clinical settings for identifying patients with depression who have these high levels of inflammation. These associations also generalized to a composite inflammation factor created by combining the measures of the hsCRP, fibrinogen, and WBC. The elevated inflammation levels in depressed individuals with maltreatment history remained robust after accounting for correlated risk factors, such as depression recurrence, low socioeconomic status in childhood or adulthood, poor health, or smoking. These results suggest that a history of childhood maltreatment may help to identify subgroups of individuals with elevated inflammation levels who are thus at risk for developing subsequent cardiovascular diseases.

In summary, the set of research studies presented above suggests that individuals who were maltreated as children may display a stress-related elevation in inflammation levels. Follow-up studies in other samples observed that this elevation in inflammation levels had likely already started during childhood (Danese et al., 2011).

1.5 Clinical Implications

The research finding presented above have potential clinical implications in depression. Depression is a recurrent and potentially progressive type of illness. The yearly or 12-month prevalence of depression is 7%, whereas the lifetime prevalence of depression is 16% (Kessler et al., 2003; Solomon et al., 2000). The finding that the lifetime prevalence of depression is only about twice as much as the yearly prevalence of depression suggests that depression is a recurrent type of illness because many of the episodes contributing to the lifetime prevalence of depression are likely to originate from the same group of people. Clinical observations support this conjecture, showing that 60% of remitted patients will have recurrence in 5 years, and growing evidence shows that each new episode of depression increases the risk of recurrence and reduces the time to recurrence. Therefore, identifying groups of people who proceed to develop recurrent types of depression can contribute to the prevention of the largest health burdens related to depression.

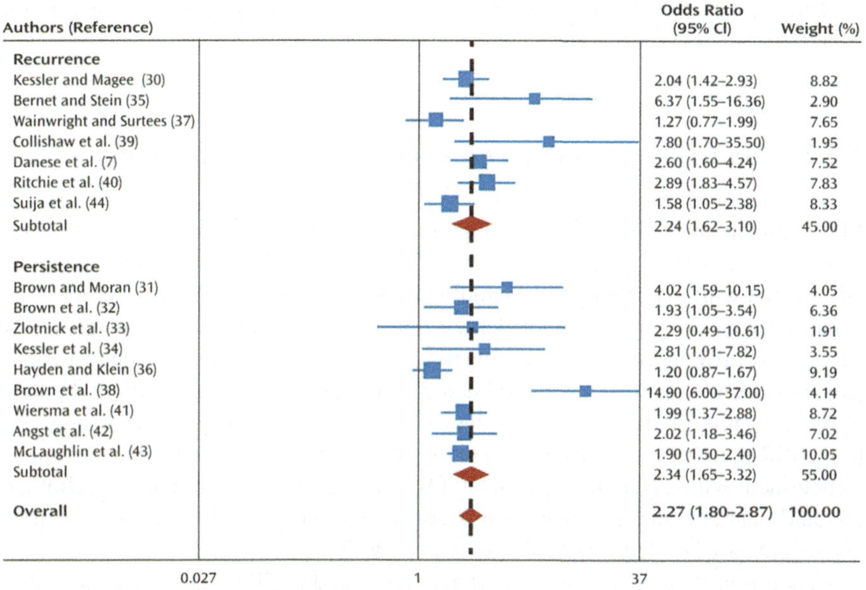

Fig. 1.2 Meta-analysis of epidemiological studies investigating the association between childhood maltreatment and depression course (random effects). The red diamonds show the combined effect sizes for studies concerned with depression recurrence and depression persistence as well as the overall effect size of the meta-analysis (top to bottom). From Nanni, V., Uher, R., & Danese, A. (2012). *American Journal of Psychiatry*, *169*, 141–151. Reprinted with permission from the American Journal of Psychiatry, (Copyright ©2012). American Psychiatric Association. All Rights Reserved

1.5.1 Childhood Maltreatment and Depression Subtypes

The different types of depression seem to have varying associations with inflammation. A large American study conducted by Ford and Erlinger (2004) found that individuals with a history of multiple recurrent cases of depression had elevated inflammation levels, while individuals with single episodes of depression did not have elevated levels compared to individuals with no depression.

If maltreatment is associated with inflammation, which is in turn associated with a recurrent subtype of depression, then one could hypothesize that maltreatment may also be related to a recurrent subtype of depression. Nanni, Uher, and Danese (2012) conducted the first meta-analysis of epidemiological studies that examined both the risk and course of depression in maltreated individuals. The researchers examined outcomes including the recurrence and the persistence of depression. Figure 1.2 presents the individual study effect sizes, error estimates, and cumulative effect size of the meta-analysis. Overall, maltreated individuals were more than twice as likely as non-maltreated controls to develop recurrent and persistent types of depression. These findings suggest that maltreatment might be associated with a specific type of depression that contributes to the large health burden related to the condition.

1.5.2 Maltreatment and Depression Treatment Outcomes

Maltreatment may also influence depression treatment outcomes. In the United Kingdom, and similarly in the United States of America, depressed adults are generally treated with psychotherapy, including cognitive behavioral therapy or interpersonal therapy, for mild cases of depression. Pharmacotherapy is used for severe cases, generally in combination with psychotherapy. In depressed young people, psychotherapy (cognitive behavioral therapy, interpersonal therapy, family therapy) is the first line of treatment regardless of depression severity. Pharmacotherapy (e.g., SSRIs) may be used in addition to psychotherapy for those who do not respond to treatment with psychotherapy alone. Overall, combined treatment—psychotherapy and pharmacotherapy together—is considered the most effective way of treating severe cases of depression (Thase et al., 1997).

Lanquillon, Krieg, Bening-Abu-Shach, and Vedder (2000) conducted a trial of amitriptyline, a tricyclic antidepressant, to patients over an eight-week period. The researchers used baseline levels of the inflammatory cytokine interleukin (IL)-6 collected prior to starting the medication to predict patient response to the treatment. The researchers found that depressed individuals who responded to pharmacological treatment had inflammation levels that were similar to those in the nondepressed control group, whereas depressed individuals who did not respond to the treatment had significantly higher levels of inflammation. This study was one of the first to support the idea that inflammation levels may affect treatment response.

If maltreatment is associated with high levels of inflammation, which is in turn associated with treatment resistance, then one could hypothesize that maltreatment may also be associated with treatment resistance in depression. Nanni et al. (2012) also presented a meta-analysis of trials of different types of treatments for depression, testing whether maltreatment could be used to identify those with unfavorable outcomes. The results, presented in Fig. 1.3, indicated that depressed patients with a history of maltreatment were, overall, more likely to respond poorly to treatment compared to depressed patients who did not have a history of maltreatment. For psychotherapy alone, no significant difference was found between depressed patients who had or had not had a history of maltreatment. For pharmacotherapy alone, an effect started to emerge, showing that depressed patients with a history of maltreatment had worse outcomes than did depressed patients without a history of maltreatment. For combined therapy, considered the most effective treatment in severe cases, the clearest effect of maltreatment emerged: depressed individuals with a history of maltreatment were almost twice as likely than depressed individu-

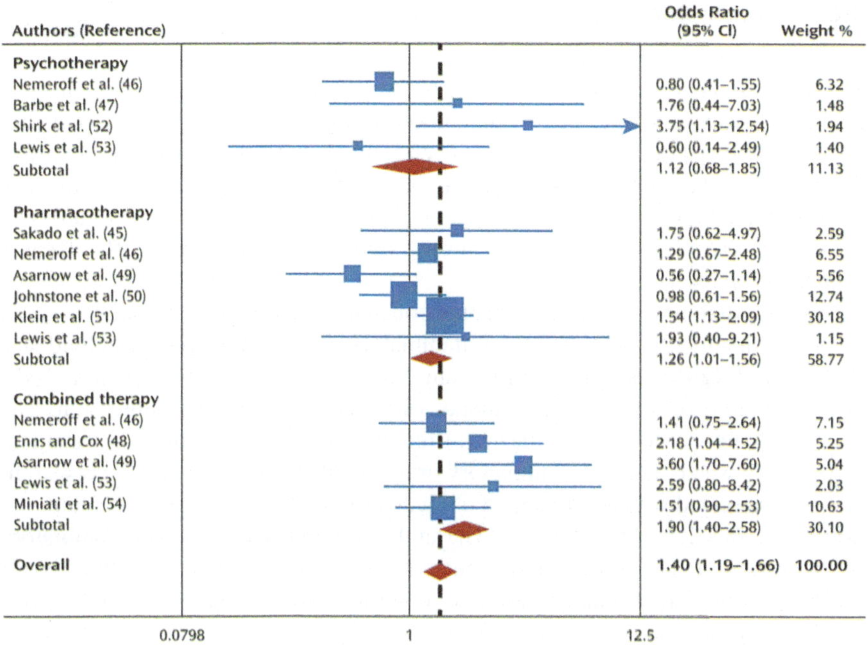

Fig. 1.3 Meta-analysis of clinical trials investigating the association between childhood maltreatment and treatment outcome of depression (fixed effects). The red diamonds show the combined effect sizes for studies concerned with psychotherapy, pharmacotherapy, and combined therapy, as well as the overall effect size of the meta-analysis (top to bottom). From Nanni, V., Uher, R., & Danese, A. (2012). *American Journal of Psychiatry*, *169*, 141–151. Reprinted with permission from the American Journal of Psychiatry, (Copyright ©2012). American Psychiatric Association. All Rights Reserved

als without a history of childood maltreatment to have poor treatment response with this form of treatment. These results suggest that more research is required to understand the pathophysiology of depression in maltreated individuals and to identify alternative pathways through which these types of depression could be treated.

In summary, maltreated children are at an elevated risk of developing a specific subtype of depression characterized by recurrent and progressive episodes of depression throughout their life course and, thus, account for a large fraction of the health burden associated with depression. Individuals who have depression and also have a history of maltreatment are at a high risk of poor response to a number of different treatments for depression. They may benefit less from combined psychotherapy and pharmacotherapy, a form of treatment considered most effective. This suggests that alternative methods of treatment need to be sought and tailored specifically to this population.

1.6 Conclusion

While researchers and clinicians have long been aware of the mental and physical health toll associated with maltreatment, knowledge about *how* maltreatment produces these types of health effects has been limited. Inflammation might be one of the pathways that contributes to these health effects. Identifying these pathways, whether inflammation or other mechanisms that may be identified in the future, will better position researchers and clinicians to explore new ways to treat difficult cases of mental illnesses.

Building upon this idea, this chapter concludes by presenting results from an intervention study that targeted the inflammatory system in depressed individuals. Raison et al. (2013) administered the anti-inflammatory drug Infliximab, a TNF-alpha inhibitor, or a placebo to patients with treatment-resistant depression. The study initially found no significant differences in the proportion of treatment response between the anti-inflammatory drug and placebo condition. The researchers then examined whether treatment efficacy differed based on baseline inflammation levels (hsCRP concentration). The authors found that the anti-inflammatory medication did not significantly benefit the patients who had low levels (CRP $\leq$ 5 mg/L) of inflammation at baseline. For patients with high levels (CRP > 5 mg/L), however, some effects started to emerge that suggest improved response with the anti-inflammatory medication. These trends will need to be examined in larger planned analysis. This study suggests that identifying those patients with depression who also have high levels of inflammation might enable clinicians to use new and effective interventions for treatment-resistant depression—anti-inflammatory compounds, for example. Maltreatment history may be one of the factors that can aid in the identification of individuals in the population, and particularly within groups of depressed individuals, who have high levels of inflammation. By targeting the specific biological vulnerabilities that are being uncovered in the population of maltreated individuals, it may be possible to adopt targeted and more effective interventions for depression.

References

Danese, A., & Baldwin, J. R. (2017). Hidden wounds? Inflammatory links between childhood trauma and psychopathology. *Annual Review of Psychology, 68*, 517–544. https://doi.org/10.1146/annurev-psych-010416-044208

Danese, A., Caspi, A., Williams, B., Ambler, A., Sugden, K., Mika, J., … Arseneault, L. (2011). Biological embedding of stress through inflammation processes in childhood. *Molecular Psychiatry, 16*(3), 244–246. https://doi.org/10.1038/mp.2010.5

Danese, A., & Lewis, S. (2017). Psychoneuroimmunology of early-life stress: The hidden wounds of childhood trauma? *Neuropsychopharmacology, 42*(1), 99–114. https://doi.org/10.1038/npp.2016.198

Danese, A., & McEwen, B. S. (2012). Adverse childhood experiences, allostasis, allostatic load, and age-related disease. *Physiology & Behavior, 106*(1), 29–39. https://doi.org/10.1016/j.physbeh.2011.08.019

Danese, A., Moffitt, T. E., Pariante, C. M., Ambler, A., Poulton, R., & Caspi, A. (2008). Elevated inflammation levels in depressed adults with a history of childhood maltreatment. *Archives of General Psychiatry, 65*(4), 409–415. https://doi.org/10.1001/archpsyc.65.4.409

Danese, A., Pariante, C. M., Caspi, A., Taylor, A., & Poulton, R. (2007). Childhood maltreatment predicts adult inflammation in a life-course study. *Proceedings of the National Academy of Sciences of the United States of America, 104*(4), 1319–1324. https://doi.org/10.1073/pnas.0610362104

Dantzer, R., O'Connor, J. C., Freund, G. G., Johnson, R. W., & Kelley, K. W. (2008). From inflammation to sickness and depression: When the immune system subjugates the brain. *Nature Reviews Neuroscience, 9*(1), 46–56. https://doi.org/10.1038/nrn2297

Ford, D. E., & Erlinger, T. P. (2004). Depression and c-reactive protein in us adults: Data from the third national health and nutrition examination survey. *Archives of Internal Medicine, 164*(9), 1010–1014. https://doi.org/10.1001/archinte.164.9.1010

Heim, C., Newport, D. J., Mletzko, T., Miller, A. H., & Nemeroff, C. B. (2008). The link between childhood trauma and depression: Insights from HPA axis studies in humans. *Psychoneuroendocrinology, 33*(6), 693–710. https://doi.org/10.1016/j.psyneuen.2008.03.008

Howren, M. B., Lamkin, D. M., & Suls, J. (2009). Associations of depression with C-reactive protein, IL-1, and IL-6: A meta-analysis. *Psychosomatic Medicine, 71*(2), 171–186. https://doi.org/10.1097/PSY.0b013e3181907c1b

Kessler, R. C., Berglund, P., Demler, O., Jin, R., Koretz, D., Merikangas, K. R., ... Wang, P. S. (2003). The epidemiology of major depressive disorder: Results from the National Comorbidity Survey Replication (NCS-R). *JAMA, 289*(23), 3095–3105. https://doi.org/10.1001/jama.289.23.3095

Kiecolt-Glaser, J. K., Preacher, K. J., MacCallum, R. C., Atkinson, C., Malarkey, W. B., & Glaser, R. (2003). Chronic stress and age-related increases in the proinflammatory cytokine IL-6. *Proceedings of the National Academy of Sciences of the United States of America, 100*(15), 9090–9095. https://doi.org/10.1073/pnas.1531903100

Lanquillon, S., Krieg, J. C., Bening-Abu-Shach, U., & Vedder, H. (2000). Cytokine production and treatment response in major depressive disorder. *Neuropsychopharmacology, 22*(4), 370–379. https://doi.org/10.1016/s0893-133x(99)00134-7

Miller, A. H., Maletic, V., & Raison, C. L. (2009). Inflammation and its discontents: The role of cytokines in the pathophysiology of major depression. *Biological Psychiatry, 65*(9), 732–741. https://doi.org/10.1016/j.biopsych.2008.11.029

Musselman, D. L., Lawson, D. H., Gumnick, J. F., Manatunga, A. K., Penna, S., Goodkin, R. S., ... Miller, A. H. (2001). Paroxetine for the prevention of depression induced by high-dose interferon alfa. *The New England Journal of Medicine, 344*(13), 961–966. https://doi.org/10.1056/nejm200103293441303

Nanni, V., Uher, R., & Danese, A. (2012). Childhood maltreatment predicts unfavorable course of illness and treatment outcome in depression: A meta-analysis. *The American Journal of Psychiatry, 169*(2), 141–151. https://doi.org/10.1176/appi.ajp.2011.11020335

Pearson, T. A., Mensah, G. A., Alexander, R. W., Anderson, J. L., Cannon, R. O., 3rd, Criqui, M., ... Vinicor, F. (2003). Markers of inflammation and cardiovascular disease: Application to clinical and public health practice: A statement for healthcare professionals from the Centers for Disease Control and Prevention and the American Heart Association. *Circulation, 107*(3), 499–511.

Raison, C. L., Rutherford, R. E., Woolwine, B. J., Shuo, C., Schettler, P., Drake, D. F., ... Miller, A. H. (2013). A randomized controlled trial of the tumor necrosis factor antagonist infliximab for treatment-resistant depression: The role of baseline inflammatory biomarkers. *JAMA Psychiatry, 70*(1), 31–41. https://doi.org/10.1001/2013.jamapsychiatry.4

Sattar, N., McConnachie, A., O'Reilly, D., Upton, M. N., Greer, I. A., Davey Smith, G., & Watt, G. (2004). Inverse association between birth weight and C-reactive protein concentrations in the

MIDSPAN family study. *Arteriosclerosis, Thrombosis, and Vascular Biology, 24*(3), 583–587. https://doi.org/10.1161/01.atv.0000118277.41584.63

Solomon, D. A., Keller, M. B., Leon, A. C., Mueller, T. I., Lavori, P. W., Shea, M. T., … Endicott, J. (2000). Multiple recurrences of major depressive disorder. *The American Journal of Psychiatry, 157*(2), 229–233. https://doi.org/10.1176/appi.ajp.157.2.229

Steptoe, A., Owen, N., Kunz-Ebrecht, S., & Mohamed-Ali, V. (2002). Inflammatory cytokines, socioeconomic status, and acute stress responsivity. *Brain, Behavior, and Immunity, 16*(6), 774–784.

Taylor, S. E., Lehman, B. J., Kiefe, C. I., & Seeman, T. E. (2006). Relationship of early life stress and psychological functioning to adult C-reactive protein in the coronary artery risk development in young adults study. *Biological Psychiatry, 60*(8), 819–824. https://doi.org/10.1016/j.biopsych.2006.03.016

Thase, M. E., Greenhouse, J. B., Frank, E., Reynolds, C. F., 3rd, Pilkonis, P. A., Hurley, K., … Kupfer, D. J. (1997). Treatment of major depression with psychotherapy or psychotherapy-pharmacotherapy combinations. *Archives of General Psychiatry, 54*(11), 1009–1015.

Whalley, L. J., & Deary, I. J. (2001). Longitudinal cohort study of childhood IQ and survival up to age 76. *BMJ, 322*(7290), 819.

Widom, C. S. (1989). The cycle of violence. *Science, 244*(4901), 160–166.

Widom, C. S., DuMont, K., & Czaja, S. J. (2007). A prospective investigation of major depressive disorder and comorbidity in abused and neglected children grown up. *Archives of General Psychiatry, 64*(1), 49–56. https://doi.org/10.1001/archpsyc.64.1.49

Chapter 2
Psychobiological Consequences of Child Maltreatment

Christine Heim

2.1 Introduction

This chapter summarizes a lecture given as part of the Third Conference of *Penn State's Child Maltreatment Solutions Network* on "New Frontiers in the Biology of Stress, Maltreatment, and Trauma." In this lecture, I discussed the lifelong programming effects of childhood adversity on disease risk and described the biological mechanisms underlying this lifelong risk. I derived implications of this knowledge on future research directions and the development of novel mechanism-informed interventions that mitigate this risk.

An unacceptably high number of children in our society are exposed to adversity while growing up. Early-life stress (ELS) encompasses exposure to various forms of severe stressors in childhood, including maltreatment, abuse, violence, neglect, and separation or loss of a parent, among other forms of ELS. It is estimated that one in five girls and boys experience some form of abuse during childhood. When other forms of ELS are considered, this number rises to nearly one in two children affected (http://www.cdc.gov/violenceprevention/acestudy/prevalence.html; Wildeman et al., 2014). The developing brain and its adaptation systems are shaped by experience, and adversity during sensitive periods of developmental plasticity can lead to profound and persistent changes in regulatory systems that leave these individuals at lifelong risk to develop a wide range of diseases and adverse developmental outcomes (Anacker, O'Donnell, & Meaney, 2014; Lupien,

Prepared for: Proceedings of the Third Conference of the *Penn State Child Maltreatment Solutions Network*. New Frontiers in the Biology of Stress Maltreatment and Trauma. Jennie Noll, Ph.D. (Ed.).

C. Heim (✉)
Institute of Medical Psychology, Charité—Universitätsmedizin Berlin, Berlin, Germany

Department of Biobehavioral Health, College of Health and Human Development, The Pennsylvania State University, University Park, PA, USA
e-mail: christine.heim@charite.de

© Springer International Publishing AG, part of Springer Nature 2018
J. G. Noll, I. Shalev (eds.), *The Biology of Early Life Stress*, Child Maltreatment Solutions Network, https://doi.org/10.1007/978-3-319-72589-5_2

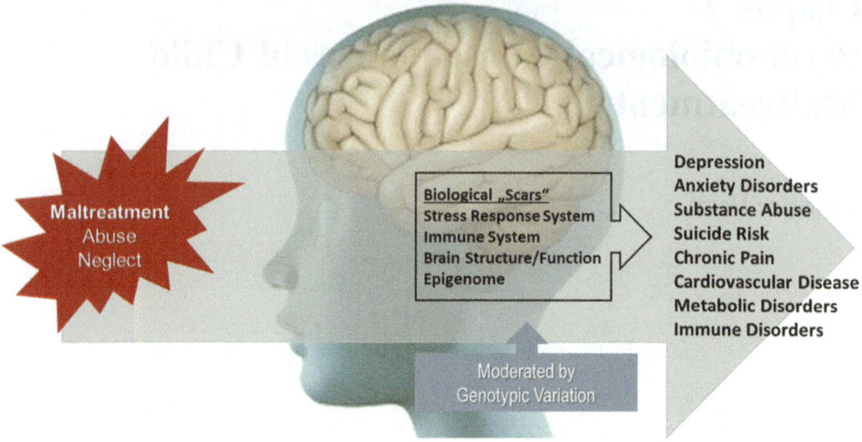

Fig. 2.1 Long-term consequences of child maltreatment

McEwen, Gunnar, & Heim, 2009a). Indeed, there is substantial evidence from epidemiological and clinical studies suggesting that exposure to ELS not only strongly and robustly increases the risk for developing psychiatric diseases, including depression and anxiety disorders and impaired cognitive development, but that it also induces lifelong risk for chronic physical disease outcomes, including cardiovascular disease, obesity, diabetes, lung cancer, chronic pain, headaches, and immune-related diseases, resulting in reduced longevity (Norman et al., 2012; Shonkoff et al., 2012). Recent evidence suggests that ELS-associated risk can be transmitted into the next generation, thus multiplying the number of affected individuals (Provençal & Binder, 2015). Indeed, the CDC estimates a $124 billion aggregate lifetime economic burden incurred by victims of child maltreatment in the USA (Fang, Brown, Florence, & Mercy, 2012), surpassing the combined economic costs of all other major pediatric health problems, including autism, asthma, pediatric cancers, exposure to environmental toxins, and obesity.

Many of the aforementioned disorders often coincide in victims of ELS and are elicited or aggravated by acute stress. Indeed, individuals with ELS appear to have decreased thresholds for exhibiting symptoms upon even mild challenges (Hammen, Henry, & Daley, 2000), and such clinical insights point to the fact that persistent sensitization of biological adaptation systems to stress may be a core mechanism that contributes to a heightened risk for a broad range of diseases across the lifespan after ELS exposure. Accordingly, studies in adults have revealed marked changes as a function of ELS exposure in stress-regulatory systems, including the endocrine, autonomic, and immune systems, as well as at the neural and molecular levels, indicating that these changes converge into heightened disease risk. Variation in genes that are relevant to stress regulation appears to moderate the effects of ELS on these biological systems, leading to differential risk versus resilience of developing clinical disorders after ELS (see Fig. 2.1).

2.2 Neurobiological Consequences of ELS

As noted above, the enduring effects of ELS on heightened disease risk are likely mediated by developmental programming effects that shape neurobiological systems during periods of heightened plasticity throughout early life. Such developmental programming may lead to persistent changes in the set-point of stress response systems and the ability of the brain and organism to adapt or compensate in response to additional challenge, which ultimately might set the stage for the development of stress-related disorders.

Our group has conducted a series of clinical studies to test this general hypothesis in humans exposed to child maltreatment. Several of these studies included depressed patients and controls, stratified by histories of early childhood maltreatment, in order to disentangle the effects of clinical diagnosis from the effects of the risk factor of ELS on neurobiological systems. We employed a standardized psychosocial laboratory stressor, the Trier Social Stress Test (TSST), which consists of a public speaking and mental arithmetic task and that reliably induces activation of the hypothalamic-pituitary-adrenal (HPA) axis and the sympathetic stress response (Heim et al., 2000). Women with a history of child abuse, without and with current major depression, exhibited markedly increased adrenocorticotropin (ACTH) responses to stress compared with controls (Heim et al., 2000). Net ACTH response was more than sixfold greater in abused women with current major depression than in controls. These women also demonstrated increased cortisol and heart rate responses to psychosocial stress. Of note, depressed women without ELS exposure demonstrated normal neuroendocrine responses, suggesting that there might be biologically distinct subtypes of depression as a function of ELS (Heim et al., 2000). Abused women who were not currently depressed exhibited normal cortisol responses, despite of their increased ACTH response, perhaps suggesting adrenal adaptation to central sensitization as a marker of current resilience in these women. Because cortisol has important regulatory effects on the central CRH and noradrenergic systems, it may be suggested that relatively decreased availability of cortisol might facilitate disinhibition of central stress responses when these women are exposed to further trauma or severe stress, eventually promoting the development of symptoms of depression through CRH effects in extra-hypothalamic circuits. These findings, taken together, suggest that sensitization of the endocrine and autonomic stress responses, presumably due to hypersecretion of central corticotropin-releasing hormone (CRH), may be a persistent consequence of ELS in humans that may contribute to the risk for psychopathology in adulthood. Of note, the effects of ELS were preserved when additionally controlling for adulthood traumas and major life events in the past year (Heim et al., 2002). Our findings were replicated in other human studies and are concordant with results from animal models of ELS, (Meaney, 2001; Rao, Hammen, Ortiz, Chen, & Poland, 2008) although there are also reports of decreased cortisol responses to stress after ELS (Carpenter, Shattuck, Tyrka, Geracioti, & Price, 2011).

As noted above, disinhibition of central CRH and noradrenergic stress response systems after ELS might contribute to heightened stress reactivity after ELS. Such disinhibition could be the result of changes in glucocorticoid-mediated feedback control of the HPA axis. In other words, if receptors for glucocorticoids in the brain were relatively resistant, one would expect enhanced neuroendocrine and autonomic stress responses as well as behavioral changes reminiscent of depression and anxiety, mediated in extra-hypothalamic CRH circuits. Therefore, consideration of glucocorticoid-mediated feedback under conditions of challenge might be particularly relevant to understand altered stress reactivity after ELS and its contribution to depression and other disorders. The combined dexamethasone/CRH test was developed as a standardized test to assess the capability of the HPA axis to maintain feedback control under challenge (Heuser, Yassouridis, & Holsboer, 1994). For this test, a high dose of dexamethasone is administered per oral in the evening, which results in shutting down of the HPA axis; the next day, CRH is injected to simulate a challenge. In healthy individuals, the HPA axis remains relatively contained in this test, reflecting functional negative feedback; however, in depressed patients, a characteristic "escape" of the HPA axis from suppression can be observed, reflecting impaired negative feedback inhibition of the HPA axis. The test is a sensitive measure of HPA axis hyperactivity in depression and further possesses the sensitivity to detect familial risk in asymptomatic first-degree relatives of depressed patients (Heuser et al., 1994; Holsboer, Lauer, Schreiber, & Krieg, 1995). We tested whether ELS exposure is related to "escape" of the HPA axis in the dexamethasone/CRH test in depressed patients. We observed markedly increased ACTH and cortisol responses to dexamethasone/CRH administration in adult men with histories of ELS and current depression, as compared to controls and depressed men without ELS (Heim, Mletzko, Purselle, Musselman, & Nemeroff, 2008). Abused men without ELS also showed increased responsiveness. The severity of the abuse predicted the degree of escape of the HPA axis in this pharmacological challenge test (Heim, Mletzko, et al., 2008). Our results suggest that ELS indeed is associated with impaired glucocorticoid-mediated feedback control of the HPA axis, which plausibly contributes to increased stress reactivity and symptoms of depression and anxiety.

The above findings of increased endocrine and autonomic responses to psychosocial stress and impaired glucocorticoid-mediated control of the HPA axis in individuals with histories of ELS are consistent with the hypothesis that central nervous system (CNS) CRH systems should be hyperactive after ELS in humans. Indeed, we observed elevated CRH concentrations in cerebrospinal fluid (CSF) in a small sample of adult women with histories of physical abuse as well as in women who experienced both sexual and physical abuse; CSF CRH concentrations were correlated with the severity and duration of the abuse (Heim, Newport, Mletzko, Miller, & Nemeroff, 2008). We further measured concentrations of the neuropeptide oxytocin (OT) in CSF of women with histories of child maltreatment. OT has marked stress-protective and anxiolytic effects and mediates prosocial behavior, such as bonding and maternal care behavior (Heim et al., 2009). We found marked decreases of CSF OT concentrations in adult women with and without histories of ELS. Using validated cut-off scores for moderate-severe exposure across the five subscales for maltreatment (physical, sexual, emotional abuse; physical, emotional neglect) of the Childhood Trauma Questionnaire (Bernstein et al., 2003), we found a dose–response relationship between the number of maltreatment types that were met and the degree of decrease in CSF oxytocin levels. Emotional abuse was most predictive of decreased CSF oxytocin levels. There was an inverse relationship between CSF oxytocin concentrations and levels of anxiety in these women (Heim et al., 2009). These findings, taken together, suggest that ELS not only leads to hyperactivity of stress mediators, such as CRH, but also interferes with the development of brain systems implicated in social attachment, which may then lead to decreased resilience against stress and anxiety. Indeed, the mechanism translating early social stress into vulnerability may not simply involve changes in stress-mediating systems, but a disturbed "balance" between stress-mediating and stress-protective neural systems.

Relative glucocorticoid resistance and stress sensitization, as observed in the above studies, may further accentuate the activation of pro-inflammatory pathways, by increased induction of NFkB, resulting in elevated pro-inflammatory cytokine release in response to stress (Bierhaus et al., 2003). Accordingly, elevated cytokine responses to stress (Carpenter et al., 2010) as well as marked elevations of C-reactive protein (CRP) (Danese et al., 2008), a marker of systemic inflammation, have been reported in humans after ELS. The effects of pro-inflammatory mediators on brain structure and function can plausibly contribute to the development of depression and anxiety disorders after ELS. The role of neuroinflammation after ELS is an area that should be further investigated in future studies.

2.3 Neurostructural and Neurofunctional Changes After ELS

A connected network of brain regions implicated in stress and emotion regulation includes the hippocampus, amygdala, and frontal cortical regions (prefrontal cortex, anterior cingulate), and this network controls peripheral outflow systems through influences on the hypothalamus and autonomic centers. Our findings of increased endocrine and autonomic responsiveness to stress after ELS indeed may reflect that a primary "lesion" after ELS may be located at the neural systems level and may involve maladaptation of the aforementioned neural circuit and failure to compensate in response to challenge. Animal models have provided causal evidence for manifold changes in central stress and emotion circuits, including structural changes and altered neurotransmitter systems (Ladd et al., 2000; Meaney, 2001).

A burgeoning number of studies suggest that there is substantial plasticity of the human brain as a function of experience (Maguire et al., 2000). Although the adult brain has the capacity for neural plasticity, the developing brain is clearly more sensitive to the organizing effects of experiences compared to the adult brain. Brain regions that are implicated in the processing and regulation of stress and emotion mature during early childhood, and there are differences in developmental trajectories between regions (Lupien, McEwen, Gunnar, & Heim, 2009b). The hippocampus is fully developed by the age of 5 years, whereas the amygdala matures earlier (2–4 years), and the prefrontal cortex develops throughout childhood and adolescence and into early adulthood. Functional connectivity between regions increases throughout childhood (Lupien et al., 2009b; Teicher, Samson, Anderson, & Ohashi, 2016). During these times of plasticity, ELS may directly impact on the development of these brain regions through experience-dependent plasticity. In addition, elevations of cortisol or inflammatory cytokines that occur as a function of ELS may exert neurotoxic effects on these structures during development and across the lifespan (Lupien et al., 2009b; Teicher et al., 2016).

The hippocampus has been the subject of intense inquiry in relation to ELS. The hippocampus exerts important inhibitory regulation of the HPA axis and plays a critical role in contextual aspects of fear conditioning. Moreover, the hippocampus is one of the most plastic regions within the CNS, with a high degree of synaptic plasticity and neurogenesis occurring in adulthood. The hippocampus has a high density of GR and is therefore particularly vulnerable to the effects of stress (Lupien et al., 2009b; Teicher et al., 2016). A large number of experimental animal studies have shown that stress and/or prolonged exposure to glucocorticoids affect the hippocampus, resulting in decreased neuronal excitability, dendritic atrophy, and apoptosis, particularly in the CA3 region, and decreased neurogenesis in the dentate gyrus (Lupien et al., 2009b). A small hippocampus is a cardinal feature of major depression (Lupien et al., 2009b; Teicher et al., 2016). Several studies of adults have now repeatedly demonstrated small hippocampal volumes after ELS (Frodl, Reinhold, Koutsouleris, Reiser, & Meisenzahl, 2010; Stein, Koverola, Hanna, Torchia, & McClarty, 1997; Teicher et al., 2016; Teicher, Anderson, & Polcari, 2012; Vythilingam et al., 2002), although studies in children are less clear (De Bellis, Hooper, Woolley, & Shenk, 2010). Our group has scrutinized the contribution of ELS to hippocampal volume loss in major depression. By stratifying depressed women into those with and without histories of ELS, we demonstrated that hippocampal volume reduction was limited to those depressed patients who were exposed to ELS, whereas depressed women without ELS exhibited normal hippocampal volume (Vythilingam et al., 2002). This result was in remarkable parallel to neuroendocrine findings and suggests that MDD in the context of ELS has a distinct pathophysiology with changes in stress-mediating systems that likely reflect a risk of developing depression in response to stress. To date, most of the studies measured the whole hippocampal volume; however, different subfields within the hippocampus are known to differ in terms of their sensitivity to stress and their role in regulating the neuroendocrine stress response. Therefore, it is crucial to use high-resolution imaging methods to investigate region-specific effects of ELS. Notably, using high-resolution hippocampal imaging, Teicher et al. (2012) reported that childhood maltreatment was strongly associated with a volume reduction in the CA3 region, the dentate gyrus, and the left subiculum. Hence, volume loss as a function of the severity of ELS indeed occurred precisely in the subfields that are sensitive to stress and glucocorticoids.

Other neuroimaging studies suggest structural and/or functional changes in the prefrontal cortex as a consequence of ELS. The PFC mediates executive functions and the regulation of goal-directed behavior and is further involved in the inhibition of impulses and emotional regulation. In particular, the medial PFC is relevant for emotional regulation, via connections with the cingulate cortex and the amygdala. The PFC also exerts inhibitory actions via indirect pathways on the HPA axis (Ulrich-Lai & Herman, 2009). Small volumes of the PFC as well as reduced blood flow in the medial PFC have been reported as features of major depression and PTSD (Ressler & Mayberg, 2007). A decreased volume of PFC areas, including the medial PFC and anterior cingulate cortex, is a consistent finding in adults with histories of ELS (Andersen et al., 2008; Frodl et al., 2010; Heim, Mayberg, Mletzko, Nemeroff, & Pruessner, 2013; Tomoda et al., 2009; Treadway et al., 2009; van Harmelen et al., 2010). In addition, ELS has been associated with structural and functional changes of the amygdala. The amygdala is a small structure in the medial temporal lobe that plays a critical role in evaluating potentially threatening information, fear conditioning, emotional processing, and memory for emotional events (Ulrich-Lai & Herman, 2009). The amygdala exerts stimulating effects on the HPA axis via indirect projections (Ulrich-Lai & Herman, 2009). It may be particularly vulnerable to the programming effects of early experience due to a high density of GR and a postnatal developmental trajectory characterized by growth and increasing connectivity until early adolescence. Studies investigating the effects of ELS on amygdala volume in humans have provided mixed findings (Tottenham et al., 2010). However, prolonged institutional rearing characterized by severe deprivation has been associated with greater amygdala volume in these children (Tottenham et al., 2010; Tottenham & Sheridan, 2009). Functional neuroimaging studies indicate that ELS is associated with sustained hyperactivity of the amygdala in response to emotionally threatening stimuli (Dannlowski et al., 2012; Grant et al., 2014; Grant, Cannistraci, Hollon, Gore, & Shelton, 2011; Tottenham et al., 2011). This sensitization of the amygdala is also apparent in response to subliminally presented stimuli (Dannlowski et al., 2013). In addition, decreased structural and functional connectivity between the medial PFC and the amygdala has been reported after ELS (Govindan, Behen, Helder, Makki, & Chugani, 2010; Grant et al., 2014). A seminal longitudinal study, following children from birth into young adulthood, found that impaired functional connectivity between the prefrontal cortex and the amygdala in young adulthood was observed as a function of ELS and was best predicted by the glucocorticoid levels of these children when they were 4.5 years old (Burghy et al., 2012). This association was significant for girls but not for boys. These findings suggest the existence of sensitive periods and sex differences in the consequences of ELS. Taken together, these findings provide convincing evidence that ELS is associated with increased reactivity of the amygdala in humans as well as reduced functional connectivity between the PFC and the amygdala, potentially contributing to a loss of "top down" control of emotional responses, which may then lead to increased physiological stress responses and risk for disorders.

More recently, an impact of ELS has also been described for sensory processing that is implicated in the perception and processing of abuse. It is well known since the seminal work of Hubel and Wiesel (Wiesel & Hubel, 1963) that visual input during a sensitive period early in life is critical for normal development of the visual cortex and vision. Cortical plasticity during sensitive periods may also account for long-term effects of enriching sensory early experiences. For example, an enlarged representation of the left hand has been observed in musicians playing a string instrument as a function of the age in childhood when they started to play (Elbert, Pantev, Wienbruch, Rockstroh, & Taub, 1995). Similar principles may apply to the effects of early adverse sensory experiences. Extending the cortical competition hypothesis, we hypothesized that if an early experience is highly aversive and developmentally inappropriate, instead of the experience enriching the brain, the brain may instead narrow its cortical representation to limit detrimental effects (Heim et al., 2013). Accordingly, using whole mantle cortical thickness analysis in adults, we observed that different forms of child maltreatment were associated with highly specific regional cortical thinning in precisely those representation areas that are implicated in the processing of each type of abuse. More specifically, we observed pronounced cortical thinning of the somatosensory genital field as a function of childhood sexual abuse. Along the same lines, emotional abuse was specifically associated with cortical thinning in the precuneus, a region that is relevant for self-awareness and self-evaluation, as well as thinning in the anterior cingulate cortex, which is relevant for emotional regulation (Heim et al., 2013). Of note, Teicher and colleagues reported similar findings for other sensory modalities, including thinning of the visual cortex after witnessing domestic violence and thinning of the auditory cortex after verbal abuse (Tomoda et al., 2011; Tomoda, Polcari, Anderson, & Teicher, 2012). These findings suggest that experience-dependent plasticity leads to effects of ELS on sensory processing areas in a highly regionally specific manner. This specific cortical thinning in sensory and processing areas may represent the most adaptive and protective response of the developing brain that may "shield" the child living under these conditions from the abusive experience, similar to sensory gating. In later life, these neuroplastic changes may represent a direct biological substrate for behavioral disorders (Heim et al., 2013).

2.4 Gene × Environment Interactions and Epigenetic Programming

Certainly, not all children exposed to ELS go on to develop depression or other stress-related disorders, even if additional stressors occur. Therefore, among other potential moderators, it is important to consider genetic factors that may convey risk for developing stress-related disorders after ELS versus genetic factors that determine resilience. Multiple studies to date have identified candidate genes in stress-regulatory systems that moderate the link between ELS and risk for depression and other disorders, including the CRH receptor 1 (CRHR1) (Bradley et al., 2008; Polanczyk et al., 2009; Ressler et al., 2010), GR (Bet et al., 2009), the GR-regulating

FK506 binding protein 5 (FKBP5) (Appel et al., 2011; Binder et al., 2008), serotonin transporter (Caspi et al., 2003; Karg, Burmeister, Shedden, & Sen, 2011), brain-derived neurotrophic factor (BDNF) (Gatt et al., 2009; Kaufman et al., 2006), and oxytocin receptor (OXTR) (Bradley, Westen, Binder, Jovanovic, & Heim, 2011) genes, among others. Gene × environment (G × E) interaction effects have also been documented at the level of intermediate phenotypes, such as neuroendocrine or amygdala reactivity (Bogdan, Williamson, & Hariri, 2012; Tyrka et al., 2009). A more recent idea is that genetic factors may reflect generally increased sensitivity to the environment, inasmuch as persons who are genetically susceptible to the detrimental effects of ELS might also be particularly amenable to the beneficial effects of a positive social environment or psychological intervention, reflecting heightened sensitivity to context or capacity for plastic change (Pluess & Belsky, 2013). Insight into G × E interactions is critically important to derive pre-disease markers to identify cases that are vulnerable to the pathogenic effects of ELS and need intervention. Genetic markers may also be used to identify cases that are susceptible to respond to a specific intervention by targeting specific systems.

A major research question in the field of ELS research concerns the molecular mechanism by which an early environmental exposure or experience can interact with a given DNA allele sequence to produce a vulnerable neurobiological phenotype with altered vulnerability for stress and disease. In this context, much attention has been directed towards epigenetic processes that may underlie the long-term consequences of ELS. Epigenetic programming refers to processes by which the environment regulates DNA transcriptional activity without altering the DNA sequence. Epigenetic changes are produced by DNA (de-) methylation, histone modifications, and non-coding RNAs (Jaenisch & Bird, 2003; Ptak & Petronis, 2010). Of these epigenetic processes, DNA (de-) methylation has been studied most extensively in relation to ELS. Specifically, DNA methylation refers to the addition of methyl groups to cytosines in cytosine-guanine (CpG) dinucleotides, which reduces the access of transcription factors to regulatory elements of the DNA, leading to transcriptional repression by decreasing binding of specific transcriptional enhancers (Jaenisch & Bird, 2003; Ptak & Petronis, 2010). Specific methyl CpG-binding domain (MBD) proteins bind to methylated DNA and interact with histone deacetylases as well as DNA methyltransferases to produce silencing of the gene and to stabilize DNA methylation status (Jaenisch & Bird, 2003; Ptak & Petronis, 2010). Conversely, demethylation and removal of MBD proteins leads to increased gene activity. Several studies in animal models and humans have now shown that ELS induces epigenetic alterations in stress-relevant genes that lead to changes in gene expression and, ultimately, a vulnerable neurobiological phenotype with increased risk for disorders. In both rodents and humans, ELS has been associated with hypermethylation of DNA sequences in the gene encoding for the GR. In a rodent model, Weaver et al. (2004) observed increased DNA methylation in a neuron-specific promoter region of the GR gene in hippocampal tissue of offspring of mothers that exhibited low maternal care behavior compared to offspring of mothers showing high maternal care behavior. This hypermethylation was associated with a decrease of NGFI-A transcription factor binding and decreased GR mRNA expression. In a post-mortem study of suicide victims, reported histories of childhood abuse were associated with the same DNA hypermethylation in the GR gene in hippocampal tissue as well as with decreases in NGFI-A binding and increases in GR mRNA expression (McGowan et al., 2009). Similar hypermethylation of the GR gene as a correlate of ELS was measured in leukocytes of healthy subjects (Tyrka, Price, Marsit, Walters, & Carpenter, 2012). Epigenetic changes have also been reported for other genes relevant to stress regulation in rodent models, including genes that regulate the expression of arginine vasopressin (Murgatroyd et al., 2009) and BDNF (Roth, Lubin, Funk, & Sweatt, 2009). In humans, a genome-wide study of promoter methylation in the hippocampal tissue of suicides revealed differential methylation of 362 genes in association with ELS, particularly genes involved in cellular or neural plasticity (Labonté et al., 2013). ELS-related differences in genome-wide methylation patterns are also seen in leukocytes from humans and are associated with changes in gene expression (Mehta et al., 2013). Taken together, both methylation and demethylation of genes involved in regulating stress responses and neural plasticity have been reported as a consequence of ELS.

More recently, Klengel et al. (2013) have provided the first evidence of a molecular pathway underlying G × E interactions after ELS by mapping a precise cascade of events that leads from ELS exposure to affective disorders via glucocorticoid-induced and genotype-directed epigenetic effects. We demonstrate that a functional polymorphism altering chromatin interaction between the transcription start site and long-range enhancers in the FKBP5 gene, an important regulator of the stress hormone system, increases the risk of developing affective disorders in adulthood by allele-specific, ELS-dependent DNA demethylation in functional glucocorticoid response elements (GREs) of FKBP5. This demethylation leads to increased stress-induced gene transcription followed by long-term dysregulation of the stress hormone system and a global impact on the function of immune cells and brain areas associated with stress regulation in risk allele carriers. FKBP5 demethylation in blood cells is correlated with ELS but not with current cortisol levels or adult trauma. Experiments in human hippocampal progenitor cells showed that a long-term demethylation of the same CpGs occurs after GR activation, suggesting that these effects could also extend to brain cells. In addition, this demethylation was only seen in proliferating and differentiating neurons, but not in mature neurons, further evidencing that this is a developmental event (Klengel et al., 2013). However, to date no study has mapped the glucocorticoid-induced epigenetic embedding of ELS in children and its subsequent effects on stress-regulatory systems and behavior. Identifying immediate temporal trajectories of this molecular mechanism, as well as G × E effects directing this molecular embedding, is essential for designing novel intervention strategies and for selecting cases for whom such interventions might be beneficial.

2.5 Current Research Needs and Implications for Intervention

Taken together, there have been substantial advances in understanding the biological mechanisms that translate exposure to ELS into lifelong risk for a broad range of diseases. It appears that ELS, in the genetically vulnerable individual, leads to a cascade of events that underlies the biological embedding of ELS and leads to phenotypic vulnerability to stress with a long-term impact on the development of disease. Biological embedding of ELS likely involves glucocorticoid-induced epigenetic modifications in stress-regulatory genes, with subsequent dysregulation of stress response systems, metabolic dysregulation, and inflammation, leading to structural and functional changes in brain regions critical for stress, emotion, and homeostatic regulation, and these trajectories likely underlie adverse mental and physical health outcomes.

However, human research on the lifelong programming effects of ELS on disease risk has mostly been limited to cross-sectional, short-term, or adult retrospective study designs, not allowing for causal inferences. Cross-sectional studies do not allow for identification of the developmental trajectories of biological embedding of ELS over time, nor do they inform about sensitive periods for the effects of ELS. While a handful of longitudinal studies exist, e.g., the E-Risk (http://www.scopic.ac.uk/StudiesERisk.html) and Dunedin (http://dunedinstudy.otago.ac.nz) studies, these were started decades ago and thus were not able to collect cutting-edge neurobiological or molecular data in the aftermath of ELS exposure or across development. Most studies, cross-sectional or longitudinal, did not adopt a multi-system approach. Thus, there is a dire gap of research ascertaining causality and considering complex interactions of multiple systems across levels of regulation. Because of these shortages, there is an even greater gap of translation between basic research insights into the biological and molecular mechanisms mediating the link between ELS and long-term disease risk and the use of this knowledge to develop novel diagnostic markers to identify cases at risk and cases susceptible to a specific intervention (personalized or precision medicine) or to develop novel interventions that directly target specific mechanisms of biological embedding. There is no doubt that ELS induces fundamental changes in regulatory systems at an early point in development, which programs these systems for life and into the next generation. To achieve critical translation, we must produce longitudinal cohort studies with comprehensive biological measures at baseline. This will allow us to map the mechanistic and temporal events of biological embedding and transmission of ELS and to understand interactions of risk and resilience factors with embedding and transmission trajectories. We further should test the potential of existing psychotherapeutic interventions to prevent or reverse these biological embedding trajectories and develop novel pharmacologically driven interventions that directly manipulate the biological mechanism. Such results will inform targeted strategies to mitigate the long-term adverse outcomes of ELS and "program" healthy and successful life trajectories in these children. Beyond that, this type of research will inform novel approaches that make use of developmental plasticity in order to promote optimal development, health, and longevity in all children.

Acknowledgments Dr. Heim's work is being funded by the German Ministry of Research and Education (01KR1301,01GL1743) and the National Institutes of Health (P50HD089922) as well as the Jacobs Foundation.

References

Anacker, C., O'Donnell, K. J., & Meaney, M. J. (2014). Early life adversity and the epigenetic programming of hypothalamic-pituitary-adrenal function. *Dialogues in Clinical Neuroscience, 16*(3), 321–333.

Andersen, S. L., Tomoda, A., Vincow, E. S., Valente, E., Polcari, A., & Teicher, M. H. (2008). Preliminary evidence for sensitive periods in the effect of childhood sexual abuse on regional brain development. *The Journal of Neuropsychiatry and Clinical Neurosciences, 20*, 292–301.

Appel, K., Schwahn, C., Mahler, J., Schulz, A., Spitzer, C., Fenske, K., … Grabe, H. J. (2011). Moderation of adult depression by a polymorphism in the FKBP5 gene and childhood physical abuse in the general population. *Neuropsychopharmacology, 36*, 1982–1991.

Bernstein, D. P., Stein, J. A., Newcomb, M. D., Walker, E., Pogge, D., Ahluvalia, T., … Zule, W. (2003). Development and validation of a brief screening version of the childhood trauma questionnaire. *Child Abuse & Neglect, 27*(2), 169–190.

Bet, P. M., Penninx, B. W., Bochdanovits, Z., Uitterlinden, A. G., Beekman, A. T., van Schoor, N. M., … Hoogendijk, W. J. (2009). Glucocorticoid receptor gene polymorphisms and childhood adversity are associated with depression: New evidence for a gene-environment interaction. *American Journal of Medical Genetics. Part B, Neuropsychiatric Genetics, 150B*, 660–669.

Bierhaus, A., Wolf, J., Andrassy, M., Rohleder, N., Humpert, P. M., Petrov, D., … Nawroth, P. P. (2003). A mechanism converting psychosocial stress into mononuclear cell activation. *Proceedings of the National Academy of Sciences USA, 100*(4), 1920–1925.

Binder, E. B., Bradley, R. G., Liu, W., Epstein, M. P., Deveau, T. C., Mercer, K. B., … Ressler, K. J. (2008). Association of FKBP5 polymorphisms and childhood abuse with risk of posttraumatic stress disorder symptoms in adults. *JAMA, 299*, 1291–1305.

Bogdan, R., Williamson, D. E., & Hariri, A. R. (2012). Mineralocorticoid receptor Iso/Val (rs5522) genotype moderates the association between previous childhood emotional neglect and amygdala reactivity. *The American Journal of Psychiatry, 169*, 515–522.

Bradley, B., Westen, D., Binder, E. B., Jovanovic, T., & Heim, C. (2011). Association between childhood maltreatment and adult emotional dysregulation: Moderation by oxytocin receptor gene. *Development and Psychopathology, 23*, 87–100.

Bradley, R., Binder, E. B., Epstein, M. P., Tang, Y., Nair, H. P., Liu, W., & Ressler, K. J. (2008). Influence of child abuse on adult depression: Moderation by the corticotropin-releasing hormone receptor gene. *Archives of General Psychiatry, 65*, 190–200.

Burghy, C. A., Stodola, D. E., Ruttle, P. L., Molloy, E. K., Armstrong, J. M., Oler, J. A., … Birn, R. M. (2012). Developmental pathways to amygdala-prefrontal function and internalizing symptoms in adolescence. *Nature Neuroscience, 15*(12), 1736–1741.

Carpenter, L. L., Gawuga, C. E., Tyrka, A. R., Lee, J. K., Anderson, G. M., & Price, L. H. (2010). Association between plasma IL-6 response to acute stress and early-life adversity in healthy adults. *Neuropsychopharmacology, 35*(13), 2617–2623.

Carpenter, L. L., Shattuck, T. T., Tyrka, A. R., Geracioti, T. D., & Price, L. H. (2011). Effect of childhood physical abuse on cortisol stress response. *Psychopharmacology, 214*(1), 367–375.

Caspi, A., Sugden, K., Moffitt, T. E., Taylor, A., Craig, I. W., Harrington, H., … Poulton, R. (2003). Influence of life stress on depression: Moderation by a polymorphism in the 5-HTT gene. *Science, 301*, 386–389.

Danese, A., Moffitt, T. E., Pariante, C. M., MRCPsych, Ambler, A., Poulton, R., & Caspi, A. (2008). Elevated inflammation levels in depressed adults with a history of childhood maltreatment. *Archives of General Psychiatry, 65*, 409–415.

Dannlowski, U., Kugel, H., Huber, F., Stuhrmann, A., Redlich, R., Grotegerd, D., … Suslow, T. (2013). Childhood maltreatment is associated with an automatic negative emotion processing bias in the amygdala. *Human Brain Mapping, 34*(11), 2899–2909.

Dannlowski, U., Stuhrmann, A., Beutelmann, V., Zwanzger, P., Lenzen, T., Grotegerd, D., & Kugel, H. (2012). Limbic scars: Long-term consequences of childhood maltreatment revealed by functional and structural magnetic resonance imaging. *Biological Psychiatry, 71*(4), 286–293.

De Bellis, M. D., Hooper, S. R., Woolley, D. P., & Shenk, C. E. (2010). Demographic, maltreatment, and neurobiological correlates of PTSD symptoms in children and adolescents. *Journal of Pediatric Psychology, 35*(5), 570–577.

Elbert, T., Pantev, C., Wienbruch, C., Rockstroh, B., & Taub, E. (1995). Increased cortical representation of the fingers of the left hand in string players. *Science, 270*(5234), 305–307.

Fang, X., Brown, D. S., Florence, C. S., & Mercy, J. A. (2012). The economic burden of child maltreatment in the United States and implications for prevention. *Child Abuse & Neglect, 36*(2), 156–165.

Frodl, T., Reinhold, E., Koutsouleris, N., Reiser, M., & Meisenzahl, E. M. (2010). Interaction of childhood stress with hippocampus and prefrontal cortex volume reduction in major depression. *Journal of Psychiatric Research, 44*(13), 799–807.

Gatt, J. M., Nemeroff, C. B., Dobson-Stone, C., Paul, R. H., Bryant, R. A., Schofield, P. R., … Williams, L. M. (2009). Interactions between BDNF Val66Met polymorphism and early life stress predict brain and arousal pathways to syndromal depression and anxiety. *Molecular Psychiatry, 14*, 681–695.

Govindan, R. M., Behen, M. E., Helder, E., Makki, M. I., & Chugani, H. T. (2010). Altered water diffusivity in cortical association tracts in children with early deprivation identified with tract-based spatial statistics (TBSS). *Cerebral Cortex, 20*(3), 561–569.

Grant, M. M., Cannistraci, C., Hollon, S. D., Gore, J., & Shelton, R. (2011). Childhood trauma history differentiates amygdala response to sad faces within MDD. *Journal of Psychiatric Research, 45*(7), 886–895.

Grant, M. M., White, D., Hadley, J., Hutcheson, N., Shelton, R., Sreenivasan, K., & Deshpande, G. (2014). Early life trauma and directional brain connectivity within major depression. *Human Brain Mapping, 35*(9), 4815–4826.

Hammen, C., Henry, R., & Daley, S. E. (2000). Depression and sensitization to stressors among young women as a function of childhood adversity. *Journal of Consulting and Clinical Psychology, 68*, 782–787.

Heim, C., Mletzko, T., Purselle, D., Musselman, D. L., & Nemeroff, C. B. (2008). The dex/corticotropin-releasing factor test in men with major depression: Role of childhood trauma. *Biological Psychiatry, 63*, 398–405.

Heim, C., Newport, D. J., Heit, S., Graham, Y. P., Wilcox, M., Bonsall, R., … Nemeroff, C. B. (2000). Pituitary-adrenal and autonomic responses to stress in women after sexual and physical abuse in childhood. *JAMA, 284*, 592–597.

Heim, C., Newport, D. J., Mletzko, T., Miller, A. H., & Nemeroff, C. B. (2008). The link between childhood trauma and depression: Insights from HPA axis studies in humans. *Psychoneuroendocrinology, 33*, 693–710.

Heim, C., Newport, D. J., Wagner, D., Wilcox, M. M., Miller, A. H., & Nemeroff, C. B. (2002). The role of early adverse experience and adulthood stress in the prediction of neuroendocrine stress reactivity in women: A multiple regression analysis. *Depression and Anxiety, 15*(3), 117–125.

Heim, C., Young, L. J., Newport, D. J., Mletzko, T., Miller, A. H., & Nemeroff, C. B. (2009). Lower CSF oxytocin concentrations in women with a history of childhood abuse. *Molecular Psychiatry, 14*, 954–958.

Heim, C. M., Mayberg, H. S., Mletzko, T., Nemeroff, C. B., & Pruessner, J. C. (2013). Decreased cortical representation of genital somatosensory field after childhood sexual abuse. *The American Journal of Psychiatry, 170*(6), 616–623.

Heuser, I., Yassouridis, A., & Holsboer, F. (1994). The combined dexamethasone/CRH test: A refined laboratory test for psychiatric disorders. *Journal of Psychiatric Research, 28*(4), 341–356.

Holsboer, F., Lauer, C. J., Schreiber, W., & Krieg, J. C. (1995). Altered hypothalamic-pituitary-adrenocortical regulation in healthy subjects at high familial risk for affective disorders. *Neuroendocrinology, 62*(4), 340–347.

Jaenisch, R., & Bird, A. (2003). Epigenetic regulation of gene expression: How the genome integrates intrinsic and environmental signals. *Nature Genetics, 33*(Suppl), 245–254.

Karg, K., Burmeister, M., Shedden, K., & Sen, S. (2011). The serotonin transporter promoter variant (5-HTTLPR), stress, and depression meta-analysis revisited: Evidence of genetic moderation. *Archives of General Psychiatry, 68*, 444–454.

Kaufman, J., Yang, B. Z., Douglas-Palumberi, H., Grasso, D., Lipschitz, D., Houshyar, S., ... Gelernter, J. (2006). Brain-derived neurotrophic factor-5-HTTLPR gene interactions and environmental modifiers of depression in children. *Biological Psychiatry, 59*, 673–680.

Klengel, T., Mehta, D., Anacker, C., Rex-Haffner, M., Pruessner, J. C., Pariante, C. M., ... Binder, E. B. (2013). Allele-specific FKBP5 DNA demethylation mediates gene-childhood trauma interactions. *Nature Neuroscience, 16*(1), 33–41.

Labonté, B., Suderman, M., Maussion, G., Lopez, J. P., Navarro-Sánchez, L., Yerko, V., ... Turecki, G. (2013). Genome-wide methylation changes in the brains of suicide completers. *The American Journal of Psychiatry, 170*(5), 511–520.

Ladd, C. O., Huot, R. L., Thrivikraman, K. V., Nemeroff, C. B., Meaney, M. J., & Plotsky, P. M. (2000). Long-term behavioral and neuroendocrine adaptations to adverse early experience. *Progress in Brain Research, 122*, 81–103.

Lupien, S., McEwen, B. S., Gunnar, M., & Heim, C. (2009a). Effects of stress throughout the lifespan on the brain, behaviour and cognition. *Nature Reviews Neuroscience., 10*(6), 434–445.

Lupien, S. J., McEwen, B. S., Gunnar, M. R., & Heim, C. (2009b). Effects of stress throughout the lifespan on the brain, behaviour and cognition. *Nature Reviews Neuroscience, 10*, 434–445.

Maguire, E. A., Gadian, D. G., Johnsrude, I. S., Good, C. D., Ashburner, J., Frackowiak, R. S., & Frith, C. D. (2000). Navigation-related structural change in the hippocampi of taxi drivers. *Proceedings of the National Academy of Sciences of the United States of America, 97*(8), 4398–4403.

McGowan, P. O., Sasaki, A., D'Alessio, A. C., Dymov, S., Labonté, B., Szyf, M., ... Meaney, M. J. (2009). Epigenetic regulation of the glucocorticoid receptor in human brain associates with childhood abuse. *Nature Neuroscience, 12*, 342–348.

Meaney, M. J. (2001). Maternal care, gene expression, and the transmission of individual differences in stress reactivity across generations. *Annual Review of Neuroscience, 24*, 1161–1192.

Mehta, D., Klengel, T., Conneely, K. N., Smith, A. K., Altmann, A., Pace, T. W., ... Binder, E. B. (2013). Type of trauma matters: Childhood maltreatment is associated with distinct genomic and epigenetic profiles in posttraumatic stress disorder. *Proceedings of the National Academy of Sciences of the United States of America, 110*(20), 8302–8307.

Murgatroyd, C., Patchev, A. V., Wu, Y., Micale, V., Bockmühl, Y., Fischer, D., ... Spengler, D. (2009). Dynamic DNA methylation programs persistent adverse effects of early-life stress. *Nature Neuroscience, 12*(12), 1559–1566.

Norman, R. E., Byambaa, M., De, R., Butchart, A., Scott, J., & Vos, T. (2012). The long-term health consequences of child physical abuse, emotional abuse, and neglect: A systematic review and meta-analysis. *PLoS Medicine, 9*(11), e1001349.

Pluess, M., & Belsky, J. (2013). Vantage sensitivity: Individual differences in response to positive experiences. *Psychological Bulletin, 139*(4), 901–916.

Polanczyk, G., Caspi, A., Williams, B., Price, T. S., Danese, A., Sugden, K., ... Moffitt, T. E. (2009). Protective effect of CRHR1 gene variants on the development of adult depression following childhood maltreatment: Replication and extension. *Archives of General Psychiatry, 66*, 978–985.

Provençal, N., & Binder, E. B. (2015). The effects of early life stress on the epigenome: From the womb to adulthood and even before. *Experimental Neurology, 268*, 10–20.

Ptak, C., & Petronis, A. (2010). Epigenetic approaches to psychiatric disorders. *Dialogues in Clinic Neuroscience, 12*(1), 25–35.

Rao, U., Hammen, C., Ortiz, L. R., Chen, L. A., & Poland, R. E. (2008). Effects of early and recent adverse experiences on adrenal response to psychosocial stress in depressed adolescents. *Biological Psychiatry, 64*, 521–526.

Ressler, K., Bradley, B., Mercer, K. B., Deveau, T. C., Smith, A. K., Gillespie, C. F., ... Binder, E. B. (2010). Polymorphisms in CRHR1 and serotonin transporter loci: Gene-gene-environment interactions on depressive symptoms. *American Journal of Medical Genetics, 153B*(3), 812–824.

Ressler, K. J., & Mayberg, H. S. (2007). Targeting abnormal neural circuits in mood and anxiety disorders: From the laboratory to the clinic. *Nature Neuroscience, 10*(9), 1116–1124.

Roth, T. L., Lubin, F. D., Funk, A. J., & Sweatt, J. D. (2009). Lasting epigenetic influence of early-life adversity on the BDNF gene. *Biological Psychiatry, 65*(9), 760–769.

Shonkoff, J. P., Garner, A. S., & Committee on Psychosocial Aspects of Child and Family Health; Committee on Early Childhood, Adoption, and Dependent Care; Section on Developmental and Behavioral Pediatrics. (2012). The lifelong effects of early childhood adversity and toxic stress. *Pediatrics, 129*(1), e232–e246.

Stein, M. B., Koverola, C., Hanna, C., Torchia, M. G., & McClarty, B. (1997). Hippocampal volume in women victimized by childhood sexual abuse. *Psychological Medicine, 27*, 951–959.

Teicher, M. H., Anderson, C. M., & Polcari, A. (2012). Childhood maltreatment is associated with reduced volume in the hippocampal subfields CA3, dentate gyrus, and subiculum. *PNAS, 109*, E563–E572.

Teicher, M. H., Samson, J. A., Anderson, C. M., & Ohashi, K. (2016). The effects of childhood maltreatment on brain structure, function and connectivity. *Nature Reviews. Neuroscience, 17*(10), 652–666.

Tomoda, A., Polcari, A., Anderson, C. M., & Teicher, M. H. (2012). Reduced visual cortex gray matter volume and thickness in young adults who witnessed domestic violence during childhood. *PLoS One, 7*(12), e52528.

Tomoda, A., Sheu, Y. S., Rabi, K., Suzuki, H., Navalta, C. P., Polcari, A., & Teicher, M. H. (2011). Exposure to parental verbal abuse is associated with increased gray matter volume in superior temporal gyrus. *NeuroImage, 54*(Suppl 1), S280–S286.

Tomoda, A., Suzuki, H., Rabi, K., Sheu, Y. S., Polcari, A., & Teicher, M. H. (2009). Reduced prefrontal cortical gray matter volume in young adults exposed to harsh corporal punishment. *NeuroImage, 47*(Suppl 2), T66–T71.

Tottenham, N., Hare, T. A., Millner, A., Gilhooly, T., Zevin, J. D., & Casey, B. J. (2011). Elevated amygdala response to faces following early deprivation. *Developmental Science, 14*(2), 190–204.

Tottenham, N., Hare, T. A., Quinn, B. T., McCarry, T. W., Nurse, M., Gilhooly, T., ... Casey, B. J. (2010). Prolonged institutional rearing is associated with atypically large amygdala volume and difficulties in emotion regulation. *Developmental Science, 13*(1), 46–61.

Tottenham, N., & Sheridan, M. A. (2009). A review of adversity, the amygdala and the hippocampus: A consideration of developmental timing. *Frontiers in Human Neuroscience, 3*, 68.

Treadway, M. T., Grant, M. M., Ding, Z., Hollon, S. D., Gore, J. C., & Shelton, R. C. (2009). Early adverse events, HPA activity and rostral anterior cingulate volume in MDD. *PLoS One, 4*, e4887.

Tyrka, A. R., Price, L. H., Gelernter, J., Schepker, C., Anderson, G. M., & Carpenter, L. L. (2009). Interaction of childhood maltreatment with the corticotropin-releasing hormone receptor gene: Effects on hypothalamic-pituitary-adrenal axis reactivity. *Biological Psychiatry, 66*, 681–685.

Tyrka, A. R., Price, L. H., Marsit, C., Walters, O. C., & Carpenter, L. L. (2012). Childhood adversity and epigenetic modulation of the leukocyte glucocorticoid receptor: Preliminary findings in healthy adults. *PLoS One, 7*, e30148.

Ulrich-Lai, Y. M., & Herman, J. P. (2009). Neural regulation of endocrine and autonomic stress responses. *Nature Reviews. Neuroscience, 10*(6), 397–409.

van Harmelen, A. L., van Tol, M. J., van der Wee, N. J., Veltman, D. J., Aleman, A., Spinhoven, P., … Elzinga, B. M. (2010). Reduced medial prefrontal cortex volume in adults reporting childhood emotional maltreatment. *Biological Psychiatry, 68*, 832–838.

Vythilingam, M., Heim, C., Newport, J., Miller, A. H., Anderson, E., Bronen, R., & Douglas Bremner, J. (2002). Childhood trauma associated with smaller hippocampal volume in women with major depression. *The American Journal of Psychiatry, 159*, 2072–2080.

Weaver, I. C., Cervoni, N., Champagne, F. A., D'Alessio, A. C., Sharma, S., Seckl, J. R., … Meaney, M. J. (2004). Epigenetic programming by maternal behavior. *Nature Neuroscience, 7*(8), 847–854.

Wiesel, T. N., & Hubel, D. H. (1963). Single-cell response in striate cortex of kittens deprived of vision in one eye. *Journal of Neurophysiology, 26*, 1003–1017.

Wildeman, C., Emanuel, N., Leventhal, J. M., Putnam-Hornstein, E., Waldfogel, J., & Lee, H. (2014). The prevalence of confirmed maltreatment among US children, 2004 to 2011. *JAMA Pediatrics, 168*(8), 706–713.

Chapter 3
Toward an Adaptation-Based Approach to Resilience

Bruce J. Ellis

The title of my talk today is "Beyond Risk and Protective Factors: An Adaptation-Based Approach to Resilience" (Ellis, Bianchi, Griskevicius, & Frankenhuis, 2017). My presentation draws on this article and reflects our collaborative work.

My hope today is to live up to the analogy of children playing leapfrog, in terms of at least comparing different perspectives. That is, I'm going to talk about traditional models of cumulative risk and resilience and then contrast this with a different approach to resilience, which we call an adaptation-based approach. In presenting this new approach, I will first talk about some of the underlying theory and research, and I will conclude by discussing implications for intervention.

One of the most robust and well-established findings in the field of human development is the very strong negative effect of poverty on all kinds of cognitive and economic achievements. Whether one operationalizes low achievement in terms of lower reading and math skills, lower executive function abilities, more learning disabilities, lower scores on standard intelligence tests and scholastic tests, or greater risk of grade repetition, expulsion, or suspension from school, growing up under impoverished economic conditions puts children at risk.

Now how do we think about this negative effect? How do we understand it, and ultimately, how do we address it? The established approach is largely based on the *deficit model* of development under stress. This deficit approach to understanding the effects of early life stress on social and cognitive functioning has different names—cumulative stress, toxic stress, diathesis stress, or allostatic load—all representing somewhat different versions of the same idea. Whatever the name, the focus of the deficit approach is on impairments in learning and behavior. This approach essentially emphasizes "what's wrong with youth" who come from harsh, unpredictable environments. Implicit in this approach is the assumption that at-risk youth are somehow broken and need to be fixed.

B. J. Ellis (✉)
Department of Psychology, University of Utah, Salt Lake City, UT, USA
e-mail: bruce.ellis@psych.utah.edu

© Springer International Publishing AG, part of Springer Nature 2018

J. G. Noll, I. Shalev (eds.), *The Biology of Early Life Stress*, Child Maltreatment Solutions Network, https://doi.org/10.1007/978-3-319-72589-5_3

When I say the assumption is that these high-risk youth need to be fixed, I mean that the deficit approach suggests they need to be made better at doing things that are commonplace for low-risk children. They need to be made better at sustaining attention, better at inhibitory control, better at following rules—in short, they need to think and act more like low-risk youth. That is the deficit story.

Yet despite the well-established links between adversity and various social and health outcomes, there is also a counterpoint to these links—the large resilience literature. The resilience literature focuses on the fact that, despite the overall low achievement levels of children and youth from lower socioeconomic backgrounds, there is striking variation in the outcomes of individuals who are exposed to high adversity. Some individuals thrive, or at least beat the odds, despite their high-risk backgrounds. This fact that some children show resilient outcomes has led to a cottage industry trying to identify resilience factors, what Masten (2001, 2014) calls the short list for resilience. This short list highlights the protective factors that actually promote resilience in the face of adversity. And there are very well established resilience factors. A few examples include intelligence, problem-solving skills, supportive family, and social relationships.

In a sense, resilience research asks, what does it take to succeed? And how can we build those attributes and qualities in at-risk youth? In a nutshell, resilience research has looked at the attributes that characterize resilient youth and then looked to develop interventions that attempt to promote these attributes. Thus, some interventions attempt to build better problem-solving skills. Others attempt to foster more supportive family and social relationships, or to enhance student–teacher trust. Essentially, these interventions are trying to build resilient qualities and relationships in youth to make them more able to deal with adversity.

This approach to intervention shares the common goal of getting young people from high-risk backgrounds to act, think, and feel more like youth from low-risk backgrounds. That is, these interventions aim to enable high-risk youth to become better at things like inhibitory control and emotion regulation and less likely to use violence as a strategy to solve problems, and so on.

Now I'm going to contrast the existing resilience research with what we call an *adaptation-based approach to resilience*. Extant interventions have not tried to leverage the unique strengths and abilities that develop specifically in response to high-risk environments. Here I don't mean that we are finding a strength (resilience) factor in youth despite their having come from high-adversity backgrounds. Rather, I am asking particularly what growing up in a high-risk environment does: i.e., how does the brain adapt to growing up in a harsh or unpredictable environment? And how can we use those adaptations? This approach treats adversity as an adaptive problem that the developing child needs to solve.

From this perspective, we would ask the question: what attention, learning, memory, problem-solving, and decision-making skills are enhanced by exposure to childhood adversity? And how can we use—that is, work with instead of against—these skills to improve intervention outcomes? This is a subtly, but importantly, different approach to thinking about intervention and resilience.

Central to this approach is the *specialization hypothesis*, published by Frankenhuis and de Weerth (2013). According to this hypothesis, harsh, unpredictable environments do not exclusively impair cognition. Instead, people's minds become developmentally adapted—that is, specialized and thus enhanced—for solving problems that are ecologically relevant in stressful environments and are thus most beneficial for thriving in such environments. So the specialization hypothesis is really very much within the larger context of the developmental programming literature. It is about how the brain was designed to track and respond to important dimensions of the local environment. What is the brain detecting and encoding in that context? How is it using that information to actually change developmental trajectories to match that context?

3.1 Animal Research

The developmental programming perspective described above is quite common in research on birds and rodents (though it is not common in developmental research in humans), including much experimental work (e.g., Crino & Breuner, 2015). In birds, this experimental research typically takes two forms. Either researchers expose young birds to food restrictions, or they systematically inject or deposit glucocorticoids into their eggs during embryonic development. In any case, with birds, as in humans and other species, there is no question that, all else being equal, it is better to grow up with lots of support and resources and food than to grow up under stress, starvation, and adversity. No one is going to challenge that assumption.

Thus, when you look at birds that have been experimentally stressed, you find many negative effects (Fig. 3.1). As one would expect, you find reduced growth, impaired immunocompetence, altered HPA axis activity, impaired neurological function, and suppressed expression of sexually selected traits in adulthood, such as bird song. Yet the negative outcomes are only half the story.

The other half of the story is that when these birds are exposed to stress they also develop specific abilities, both morphologically and behaviorally, that allow them to do well under stressful conditions (Fig. 3.1; see Ellis et al., 2017, for a review). For example, in research on barn swallows, European starlings, and great tits, researchers found that individuals that are exposed to high levels of glucocorticoids during embryonic development tend to be smaller, as exposure tends to reduce growth. But these individuals also tend to be faster. They achieve faster take-off speeds, and essentially they are better at getting away from predators. They are more maneuverable. They are well adapted to a dangerous environment. You also find, for example, with Zebra finches, faster learning of a novel foraging task.

Again, the idea here is that the stress a bird is exposed to early in life actually prepares it for the environment it is going to mature into. Prenatal exposure to high levels of glucocorticoids is a signal that the bird's environment is dangerous and uncertain. Accordingly, you see learning strategies in these birds that match that type of environment, such as quicker learning of a novel foraging task and more

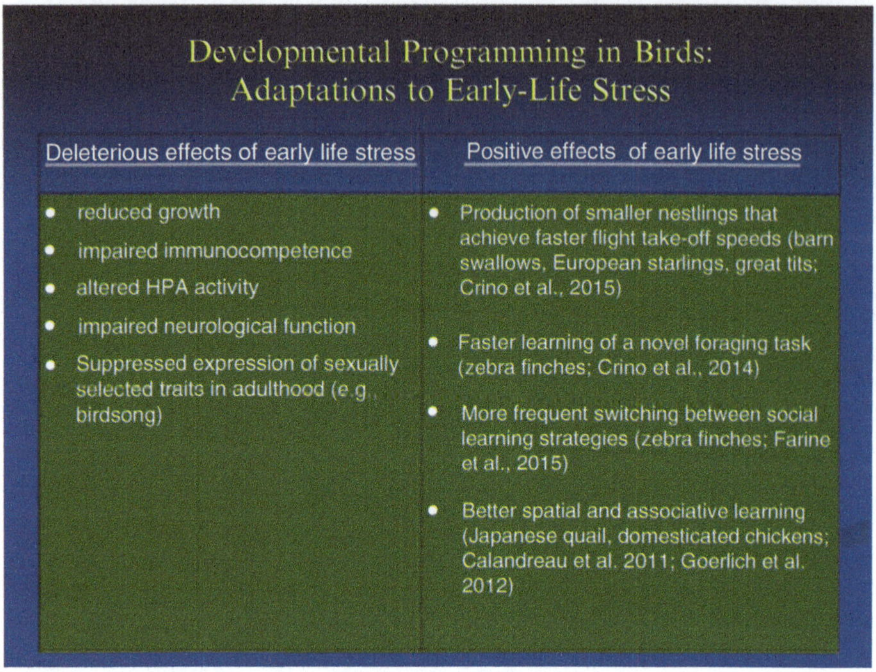

Fig. 3.1 Bivalent effects in birds of developmental exposures to early-life stress

frequent switching between different social learning strategies (Fig. 3.1). Such birds are more likely to stop one strategy and try another when it is not working, which is somewhat akin to task switching. You also find in Japanese quail and domesticated chickens, better spatial and associative learning. The finding of associative learning is particularly interesting, because it involves monitoring contingencies in your environment, which should be especially relevant in an unpredictable, uncertain context.

Moving on from birds to rodents, there is also well-established rodent literature on this topic, particularly the work of our neuroscience colleagues, Michael Meaney, Francis Champagne, Nicole Cameron, and Darlene Francis (Cameron et al. 2005; Champagne, Francis, Mar, & Meaney, 2003; Champagne & Meaney, 2006; Francis, Champagne, & Meaney, 2000; Frances, Diorio, Liu, & Meaney, 1999). This work has focused especially on the effects of licking and grooming in rodents. Rat mothers, like human mothers, show quite a lot of natural variation in the quality of parental investment. Some dams engage in high levels of parental care in the form of elevated levels of licking and grooming and arched-back nursing of their offspring and later weaning ages. Others show lower investment along these dimensions. Equally important but less widely talked about is that the parental investment of rats, like parental investment of humans, also tracks ecological context (reviewed in Champagne, 2008; Beery & Francis, 2011).

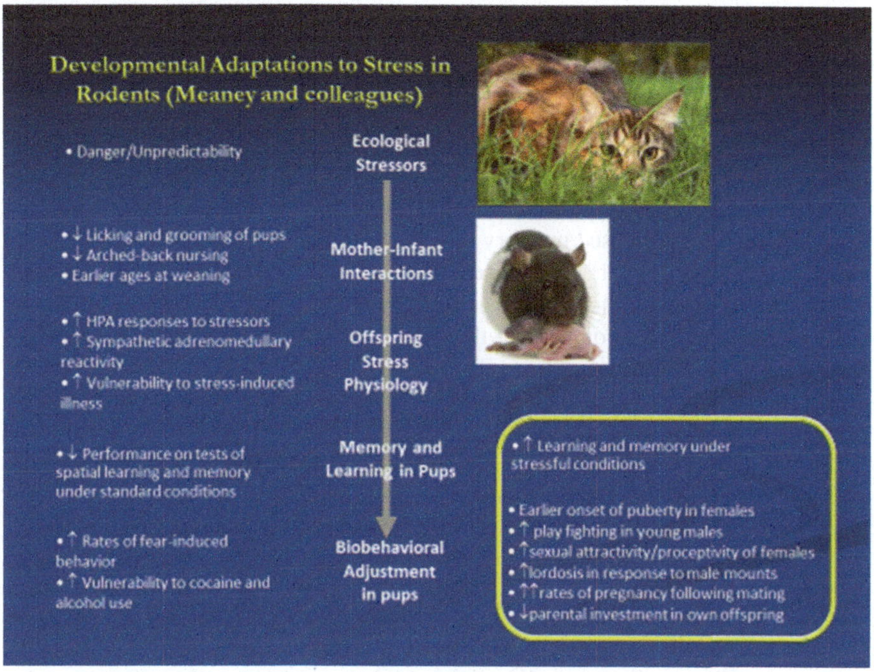
Developmental Adaptations to Stress in Rodents (Meaney and colleagues)
• Danger/Unpredictability
Ecological Stressors
• ↓ Licking and grooming of pups
• ↓ Arched-back nursing
• Earlier ages at weaning
Mother-Infant Interactions
• ↑ HPA responses to stressors
• ↑ Sympathetic adrenomedullary reactivity
• ↑ Vulnerability to stress-induced illness
Offspring Stress Physiology
• ↓ Performance on tests of spatial learning and memory under standard conditions
Memory and Learning in Pups
• ↑ Rates of fear-induced behavior
• ↑ Vulnerability to cocaine and alcohol use
Biobehavioral Adjustment in pups
• ↑ Learning and memory under stressful conditions
• Earlier onset of puberty in females
• ↑ play fighting in young males
• ↑sexual attractivity/proceptivity of females
• ↑lordosis in response to male mounts
• ↑↑rates of pregnancy following mating
• ↓parental investment in own offspring

Fig. 3.2 Bivalent effects in rodents of developmental exposure to early-life stress

Rat mothers that grow up under high ecological stress, such as high predation pressure or hunger, are much more likely to show the low licking and grooming style. In other words, when the mothers themselves are in a context where they have to devote a lot of energy to just staying alive or dealing with a suboptimal environment, there is less energy left to devote to offspring. So here in this picture (Fig. 3.2), the cat represents the ecological stressor for the rat. As is well documented in the work by Michael Meaney and colleagues, these different parenting styles (i.e., high vs. low licking and grooming) result in a variety of epigenetic changes in the offspring (Meaney, 2010). These changes are reflected in offspring stress physiology. With low licking and grooming, stress response systems are regulated toward heightened HPA responses to stressors and heightened sympathetic adrenal medullary reactivity. This in turn is associated with vulnerability to stress-induced illness. Further, under standard (low-stress) testing conditions, low licking and grooming leads to impairments of learning and memory (such as on spatial learning tasks and basic memory tasks). As you continue down the pathway and look at bio-behavioral adjustment, you see higher rates of fear-induced behavior and, when exposed to substances, more vulnerability to cocaine and alcohol use.

In total, when you look at this rat work, if you want to come at it from a deficit perspective, you can tell a deficit story. You can talk about all the bad things combining, from altered stress physiology, to poor learning and memory, to substance abuse. But that is only half the story.

The other half of the story is that those very same rats that showed impaired learning under basic, low-stress conditions (when animals are extensively habituated to testing conditions) showed enhancements when tested under high-stress conditions (Bagot et al., 2009; Champagne et al., 2008). High-stress conditions included corticosteroid treatments that mimicked high-state stress. Under such conditions, rats with a developmental history of low licking and grooming showed increased hippocampal long-term potentiation (LTP; a cellular model of learning and memory) and increased memory on a hippocampal-dependent contextual fear-conditioning task. In total, when these rats are tested under conditions that are more reminiscent of the conditions under which they grew up, they do not look impaired. They look like they are doing better than their peers that experienced high levels of licking and grooming. You also see earlier onset of puberty in these rats (Cameron et al., 2008). In general, animals that grow up under stressful and uncertain conditions where life may be short tend to go to seed early (Ellis, 2004). With guppies, if you just put the scent of a predator into their tank, it will cause pre-pubescent guppies to go through puberty more quickly. Just smelling a predator hastens their development. You see a similar result in rats that have received low maternal care.

In rats that have experienced low licking and grooming, you also see more play fighting in males (Parent & Meaney, 2008) and stronger defensive responses to an intruder (Menard & Hakvoort, 2007). In addition, you see more sexual attractivity and proceptivity in females (Cameron, Fish, & Meaney, 2008; Sakhai, Kriegsfeld, & Francis, 2011). The females that grow up with low licking and grooming mothers are just better at mating. They are better at doing ear wiggling, hopping, and darting, and the other rat mating signals, which makes them better at attracting mates. That is, they are more likely to show lordosis in response to male mounts. They also have sharply higher rates of getting pregnant following mating. They are simply much better at getting pregnant. Then they tend to show lower levels of parental investment in their own offspring.

This is not dysfunction—some kind of impaired response. These are systematic adaptive responses to growing up under uncertain conditions. Most critically, if you want to understand the deficits—if you want to understand the maladaptation, or what we often think of as dysfunction—you really have to understand these functional responses first. Because that is what happens under high-stress conditions. The negative side of the equation—the costs involved—often consists of tradeoffs inherent in these adaptive responses.

It is worth noting that this balance of the cost and benefits is also apparent in rats that are exposed to more severe stress. For example, in the work of Oomen et al. (2010), young rat pups actually experienced maternal deprivation at day three. In these young rats, they took the mother away, and the rat had to go an entire day without any maternal contact. That's a severe stressor. As you would expect, there were various negative effects of this separation, such as reduced spatial learning and neurogenesis. But once again, that finding is only half the story. The other half is that even those rats that had more severe deprivation, which is more a model for child abuse, showed improved hippocampal synaptic plasticity and emotional learning under high-stress conditions. For example, they showed enhanced contextual and cued fear conditioning.

3.2 Human Research

So what about humans? Does stress simply impair cognition? Or does stress adaptively shape cognition to match local conditions, including early life adversity? This comes back to the specialization hypothesis. Do children developing under stressful conditions become good at thinking and reasoning in certain ways? In terms of this question, the very first research that systematically addressed it, where the point or goal of the research was to test the specialization hypothesis in humans, was only published in 2015 (Mittal, Griskevicius, Simpson, Sung, & Young, 2015). In other words, this is a new area of research. However, some extant research is indirectly relevant to evaluating the specialization hypothesis. That work has mostly focused on children who have experienced significant psychosocial adversity, particularly child maltreatment. Although the goal of this work was not to look at cognitive advantages, researchers have ended up finding a few things here and there. This literature suggests that maltreated children develop enhanced abilities for detecting, learning, and remembering stimuli that are ecologically relevant to them.

Probably the most well known researcher on this topic is Seth Pollak (Pollak, 2008; Pollak, Messner, Kistler, & Cohn, 2009). He has looked at adaptation to really dangerous home environments. (Note that while I frame it as adaptation to home environments, he would probably frame it differently.) His work shows that physically abused children are highly attuned to threat-relevant information. They orient more rapidly to angry faces and angry voices. They are more accurate in identifying angry facial expressions from degraded pictures. They are also more accurate, but not faster, in identifying fearful faces. Pollak's research is consistent with the idea that, in a hostile environment, it is especially important to be able to detect and predict threats.

There is also some research about memory for negative information and events. In one study, children with histories of maltreatment were asked to recall details of a highly stressful anogenital examination received 3 days earlier, which was part of an inpatient abuse assessment. Children who had experienced greater trauma were better at identifying in a photo lineup the doctor who had examined them (Eisen, Goodman, Qin, Davis, & Crayton, 2007). However, maltreated children actually show worse photo identification accuracy of adults they interact with in a positive, playful interaction. Here again, some specific abilities were heightened in response to adversity. Maltreated children have also been found to recall a greater number of distracting, aggressive stimuli, such as swords and guns and knives, than do non-maltreated children when doing a fruit identification task (Rieder & Cicchetti, 1989).

Moving away from specific research on maltreated children and looking more at normative populations, probably the area where this topic has been studied the most is in terms of empathic accuracy. Here we find a nice body of work conducted by Kraus, Piff, Mendoza-Denton, Rheinschmidt, and Keltner (2012) based largely on community samples of adults. In this work, they show that socioeconomic adversity is linked to better empathic accuracy. Empathic accuracy means increased accuracy in the perception of other people's emotions. The underlying idea is that individuals from lower socioeconomic status (SES) backgrounds are more contextual. Enhanced empathic accuracy may promote behavioral prediction and management of external social forces and individuals that exert substantial control over one's life (which occurs chronically for people at low SES; see Kraus et al., 2012).

In one study, high school educated adults were compared with college educated adults, and researchers found that individuals with only a high school education actually did significantly better on standard tests of empathic accuracy—tests that require accurately labeling, with emotion terms, different facial expressions. Lower SES adults were also more accurate at inferring specific emotions such as contempt or sympathy from someone who was interviewing them. Finally, lower SES adults showed more physiological responses and patterns of emotional contagion that are empathically linked to those of a social interaction partner: they were more likely to match who they were interacting with. In total, individuals from higher adversity backgrounds were specifically developing certain abilities, in this case, a certain type of emotional competence.

As another example, consider variation in attachment styles, which can be roughly labeled as ranging from more secure to insecure attachments. Life history theorists have emphasized that attachment insecurity is actually quite relevant to a history of family stress and low parental investment. Among boys from low-risk families, 3-year-olds with insecure attachment histories, measured at 6 months, recalled negative events such as spilling juice seen at a puppet show more accurately than they recalled positive events such as receiving a present in the puppet show, whereas boys with secure attachment showed exactly the opposite. In total, boys with insecure attachment histories were actually superior at remembering negative things that happened in this puppet show that they saw (Belsky, Spritz, & Crnic, 1996).

Finally, let us consider one set of studies that has actually been designed from the outset to test the specialization hypothesis (Mittal et al., 2015). This study looked particularly at executive function abilities, comparing inhibitory control versus attention shifting. An important underlying idea in this research was that inhibitory control and attention shifting are adapted to different environmental contexts. When growing up in an environment that is changing and uncertain, in which one does not know what is coming, it may be advantageous to be good at attention shifting—to be able to unstick your attention from one area and change and attend to another area. This kind of shifting between different tasks should promote detection of threats and taking advantage of fleeting opportunities in chaotic/unpredictable environments. In contrast, when growing up in an environment that is stable with a predictable future, it may be more important to excel in inhibitory control and delay of gratification—to be able to focus on long-term goals and stick with what you are doing. That is because, in this predictable context, long-term goals are rewarded, as is inhibitory control, and delay of gratification may actually result in larger returns.

That was the idea behind Mittal et al.'s (2015) research. Student and community samples that experienced different levels of childhood stress and unpredictability were tested on whether they showed enhanced or diminished inhibitory control and

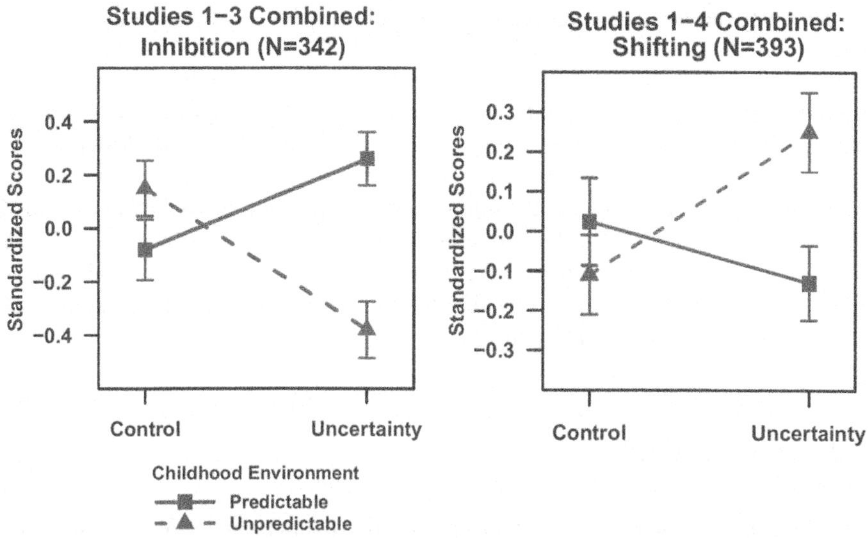

Fig. 3.3 Interactions between childhood unpredictdability and current manipulated economic uncertainty: Contrasting effects on inhibitory control and attention shifting. Reprinted from: Mittal, C., Griskevicius, V., Simpson, J. A., Sung, S., & Young, E.S. (2015). Cognitive adaptations to stressful environments: When childhood adversity enhances adult executive function. *Journal of Personality and Social Psychology*, *109*, 604–621

shifting attention. However, drawing on the animal behavior research, the researchers hypothesized that childhood adversity is most likely to influence later cognitive function when participants are currently under duress. This hypothesis was inspired by the rat research reviewed earlier in which rats that experienced high levels of early life stress were inferior under standard laboratory conditions but showed superior performance under stressful conditions.

Accordingly, this research included a psychological manipulation. The researchers randomly assigned participants to either a future economic unpredictability condition in which they saw a presentation indicating that the economy had tanked, that there would be no jobs in the future, and that things were getting worse, or a control condition in which they saw nature pictures. The dependent variables included inhibitory control and task shifting. On the left side of Fig. 3.3 are the results of the studies focusing on inhibition. Low versus high levels of childhood unpredictability (growing up in a chaotic home where people and routines changed a lot) served as the main predictor variable in this work. What you see is that under the control conditions, there were no differences in inhibitory control, but under conditions of manipulated economic uncertainty, the individuals with more predictable childhood developmental histories became better at inhibitory control, better at inhibiting dominant responses, whereas individuals who grew up in more unpredictable home environments became worse at it. This was a statistically significant difference in the uncertainty condition.

The opposite finding emerged with task shifting (Fig. 3.3). Under the manipulated economic uncertainty condition, individuals from more unpredictable home environments actually became better at task shifting, whereas individuals who grew up under more predictable conditions became worse at task shifting. This finding has now been replicated several times, as published in this report (Mittal et al., 2015). In conclusion, this is the first set of experiments demonstrating the conditions under which exposure to a childhood stress leads to improved adult cognitive functioning on a major task. Most interesting, exposure to unpredictable childhood conditions had specific and opposite effects on two major types of executive function consistent with the notion that shifting, but not inhibition, is more useful and adaptive in unpredictable environments.

3.3 Intervention

Now let's think about how to apply this perspective to intervention. We of course can think about well-known standard approaches to intervention, as captured by various metaphors. Here are some that I like. One of them is the metaphor of the cat's claws (Ellis et al., 2012) where children from high-risk backgrounds often come into school like a cat with its claws extended. They may have a hostile attribution bias, insecure attachment, and an exploitive interpersonal style. A lot of interventions are trying to get the cat to retract its claws to be more trusting, more comfortable in school, and more connected to the teacher. We can talk about other metaphors as well, such as building a better cognitive toolbox or increasing reserve capacity. Whatever metaphor you use, the standard approach is trying to get these children to essentially act, think, and feel more like children who are coming from lower risk backgrounds so they can connect with their teachers and do well in school.

However, two limitations of this approach are worth discussing. One, this intervention is trying to reprogram people, which is hard to do. We know from all that rat research that early life experiences result in epigenetic changes—that there is biological embedding of stress across multiple central neural and peripheral neuroendocrine systems. Thus, from the outset, these attempts to change individuals are fighting an uphill battle that is difficult to win. These approaches are also based on a mismatch assumption—that individuals are adapted to one environment, and now they're going into another environment in which there's a mismatch, and we need to change them.

The adaptation-based approach to resilience, advocated here, does not question the assumption that early life stress undermines certain cognitive abilities. But such well-documented deficits, focusing on "what's wrong with the kids," may again only be half the story. The other half is simply asking, "What's right with these youth?" This alternative adaptation-based approach asks: "What cognitive abilities are enhanced? What learning abilities, memory, problem-solving, and decision-making strategies are actually improved by exposure to adversity?" Then, secondly, how can we use—that is, work with instead of against—these strategies to improve intervention outcomes? How can we use them to develop better educational and job training strategies? How can we have a truly strength-based approach that really leverages what individuals are getting from high-risk environments (see extended discussion in Ellis et al. 2017)?

Here is an example that we are working on testing in my lab. We are testing the hypothesis that attentional flexibility in the form of enhanced attention shifting is linked to better contingency-based learning. That is, more attentionally flexible people contact and respond to immediate and environmental contingencies more quickly than less attentionally flexible people. If we can show that attention shifting, which is enhanced in high-risk kids, actually facilitates associative learning, then you have a path forward for using those cognitive abilities to enhance intervention and educational school outcomes for these kids.

My point in talking about these things is not to argue that one set of skills (e.g., attention shifting) is better than another set of skills (e.g., inhibitory control), but that each set of skills is adaptive in different contexts. My real point is that we need to begin studying these adaptations in context because it is a lot easier to work with them than against them. And if you work with them, then you're not creating a mismatch between what the children are doing in your intervention and what they are doing when they go back home, or when they go into work, or when they are with their friends. Instead, you are actually leveraging what they are good at.

As stress and resilience researchers, we are fundamentally interested in risk and protective factors. We are fundamentally interested in studying the darkness that faces certain children and how they emerge from that darkness. But I would also say we need to see through that darkness to leverage it for what it gives us. I want to encourage people to start thinking beyond risk and protective factors toward actual adaptations to stress.

I want to conclude this essay by posing a fundamental question that rests at the heart of the issue: Why should knowledge about the cognitive strengths of youth who are adapted to harsh, unpredictable environments, of which we know so little (with the first study published in 2015!), be any less useful than knowledge about their impairments, of which we know so much? The better we understand these cognitive adaptations to harsh environments, including the strengths of at-risk youth, the more effectively we can tailor education, policy, and interventions to fit their needs and potentials (Ellis et al., 2017).

References

Bagot, R. C., van Hasselt, F. N., Champagne, D. L., Meaney, M. J., Krugers, H. J., & Joëls, M. (2009). Maternal care determines rapid effects of stress mediators on synaptic plasticity in adult rat hippocampal dentate gyrus. *Neurobiology of Learning and Memory, 92*, 292–300. https://doi.org/10.1016/j.nlm.2009.03.004

Beery, A. K., & Francis, D. D. (2011). Adaptive significance of natural variations in maternal care in rats: A translational perspective. *Neuroscience & Biobehavioral Reviews, 35*(7), 1552–1561.

Belsky, J., Spritz, B., & Crnic, K. (1996). Infant attachment security and affective-cognitive information processing at age 3. *Psychological Science, 7*, 111–114. https://doi.org/10.1111/j.1467-9280.1996.tb00339.x

Calandreau, L., Bertin, A., Boissy, A., Arnould, C., Constantin, P., Desmedt, A., & Leterrier, C. (2011). Effect of one week of stress on emotional reactivity and learning and memory performances in Japanese quail. *Behavioural Brain Research, 217*, 104–110.

Cameron, N., Del Corpo, A., Diorio, J., McAllister, K., Sharma, S., & Meaney, M. J. (2008). Maternal programming of sexual behavior and hypothalamic-pituitary-gonadal function in the female rat. *PLoS One, 3*(5), e2210. https://doi.org/10.1371/journal.pone.0002210

Cameron, N. M., Champagne, F. A., Parent, C., Fish, E. W., Ozaki-Kuroda, K., & Meaney, M. J. (2005). The programming of individual differences in defensive responses and reproductive strategies in the rat through variations in maternal care. *Neuroscience and Biobehavioral Reveiws, 29*, 843–865.

Cameron, N. M., Fish, E. W., & Meaney, M. J. (2008). Maternal influences on the sexual behavior and reproductive success of the female rat. *Hormones and Behavior, 54*, 178–184. https://doi.org/10.1016/j.yhbeh.2008.02.013

Champagne, D. L., Bagot, R. C., van Hasselt, F., Ramakers, G., Meaney, M. J., De Kloet, E. R., … Krugers, H. (2008). Maternal care and hippocampal plasticity: Evidence for experience-dependent structural plasticity, altered synaptic functioning, and differential responsiveness to glucocorticoids and stress. *The Journal of Neuroscience, 28*, 6037–6045. https://doi.org/10.1523/jneurosci.0526-08.2008

Champagne, F. A. (2008). Epigenetic mechanisms and the transgenerational effects of maternal care. *Frontiers in Neuroendocrinology, 29*(3), 386–397.

Champagne, F. A., Francis, D. D., Mar, A., & Meaney, M. J. (2003). Variations in maternal care in the rat as a mediating influence for the effects of environment on development. *Physiology & Behavior, 79*, 359–371.

Champagne, F. A., & Meaney, M. J. (2006). Stress during gestation alters postpartum maternal care and the development of the offspring in a rodent model. *Biological Psychiatry, 59*(12), 1227–1235.

Crino, O. L., & Breuner, C. W. (2015). Developmental stress: Evidence for positive phenotypic and fitness effects in birds. *Journal of Ornithology, 156*, 389–398. https://doi.org/10.1007/s10336-015-1236-z

Crino, O. L., Driscoll, S. C., Ton, R., & Breuner, C. W. (2014). Corticosterone exposure during development improves performance on a novel foraging task in zebra finches. *Animal Behaviour, 91*, 27–32. https://doi.org/10.1016/j.anbehav.2014.02.017

Eisen, M. L., Goodman, G. S., Qin, J., Davis, S., & Crayton, J. (2007). Maltreated children's memory: Accuracy, suggestibility, and psychopathology. *Developmental Psychology, 43*, 1275–1294. https://doi.org/10.1037/0012-1649.43.6.1275

Ellis, B. J. (2004). Timing of pubertal maturation in girls: An integrated life history approach. *Psychological Bulletin, 130*, 920–958.

Ellis, B. J., Bianchi, J., Griskevicius, V., & Frankenhuis, W. E. (2017). Beyond risk and protective factors: An adaptation-based approach to resilience. *Perspectives on Psychological Science, 12*, 561–587.

Ellis, B. J., Del Giudice, M., Dishion, T. J., Figueredo, A. J., Gray, P., Griskevicius, V., … Wilson, D. S. (2012). The evolutionary basis of risky adolescent behavior: Implications for science, policy, and practice. *Developmental Psychology, 48*, 598–623. https://doi.org/10.1037/a0026220

Farine, D. R., Spencer, K. A., & Boogert, N. J. (2015). Early-life stress triggers juvenile zebra finches to switch social learning strategies. *Current Biology, 25*, 2184–2188. https://doi.org/10.1016/j.cub.2015.06.071

Francis, D. D., Champagne, F. C., & Meaney, M. J. (2000). Variations in maternal behaviour are associated with differences in oxytocin receptor levels in the rat. *Journal of Neuroendocrinology, 12*, 1145–1148.

Francis, D. D., Diorio, J., Liu, D., & Meaney, M. J. (1999). Nongenomic transmission across generations of maternal behavior and stress responses in the rat. *Science, 286*, 1155–1158.

Frankenhuis, W. E., & de Weerth, C. (2013). Does early-life exposure to stress shape or impair cognition? *Current Directions in Psychological Science, 22*, 407–412. https://doi.org/10.1177/0963721413484324

Goerlich, V. C., Nätt, D., Elfwing, M., Macdonald, B., & Jensen, P. (2012). Transgenerational effects of early experience on behavioral, hormonal and gene expression responses to acute stress in the precocial chicken. *Hormones and Behavior, 61*, 711–718. https://doi.org/10.1016/j.yhbeh.2012.03.006

Kraus, M. W., Piff, P. K., Mendoza-Denton, R., Rheinschmidt, M. L., & Keltner, D. (2012). Social class, solipsism, and contextualism: How the rich are different from the poor. *Psychological Review, 119*, 546–572. https://doi.org/10.1037/a0028756

Masten, A. S. (2001). Ordinary magic: Resilience processes in development. *American Psychologist, 56*, 227–238. https://doi.org/10.1037/0003-066x.56.3.227

Masten, A. S. (2014). *Ordinary magic: Resilience in development*. New York, NY: Guilford Press.

Meaney, M. J. (2010). Epigenetics and the biological definition of gene × environment interactions. *Child development, 81*, 41–79.

Menard, J. L., & Hakvoort, R. M. (2007). Variations of maternal care alter offspring levels of behavioural defensiveness in adulthood: Evidence for a threshold model. *Behavioural Brain Research, 176*, 302–313. https://doi.org/10.1016/j.bbr.2006.10.014

Mittal, C., Griskevicius, V., Simpson, J. A., Sung, S., & Young, E. S. (2015). Cognitive adaptations to stressful environments: When childhood adversity enhances adult executive function. *Journal of Personality and Social Psychology, 109*, 604–621. https://doi.org/10.1037/pspi0000028

Oomen, C. A., Soeters, H., Audureau, N., Vermunt, L., van Hasselt, F. N., Manders, E. M., … Krugers, H. (2010). Severe early life stress hampers spatial learning and neurogenesis, but improves hippocampal synaptic plasticity and emotional learning under high-stress conditions in adulthood. *The Journal of Neuroscience, 30*, 6635–6645. https://doi.org/10.1523/jneurosci.0247-10.2010

Parent, C. I., & Meaney, M. J. (2008). The influence of natural variations in maternal care on play fighting in the rat. *Developmental Psychobiology, 50*, 767–776. https://doi.org/10.1002/dev.20342

Pollak, S. D. (2008). Mechanisms linking early experience and the emergence of emotions: Illustrations from the study of maltreated children. *Current Directions in Psychological Science, 17*, 370–375. https://doi.org/10.1111/j.1467-8721.2008.00608.x

Pollak, S. D., Messner, M., Kistler, D. J., & Cohn, J. F. (2009). Development of perceptual expertise in emotion recognition. *Cognition, 110*, 242–247. https://doi.org/10.1016/j.cognition.2008.10.010

Rieder, C., & Cicchetti, D. (1989). Organizational perspective on cognitive control functioning and cognitive-affective balance in maltreated children. *Developmental Psychology, 25*, 382–393. https://doi.org/10.1037//0012-1649.25.3.382

Sakhai, S. A., Kriegsfeld, L. J., & Francis, D. D. (2011). Maternal programming of sexual attractivity in female long Evans rats. *Psychoneuroendocrinology, 36*, 1217–1225. https://doi.org/10.1016/j.psyneuen.2011.02.016

Frankenhuis, W. E., & de Weerth, C. (2013). Does early-life exposure to stress shape or impair cognition? *Current Directions in Psychological Science, 22*, 407–412. https://doi.org/10.1177/0963721413484324.

[illegible]

Kühn, S., [illegible]

[illegible]

Chapter 4
Developmental Traumatology: Brain Development in Maltreated Children With and Without PTSD

Jacoba Rock, Charles F. Geier, Jennie G. Noll, and Michael D. De Bellis

4.1 Introduction, Goals, and Rationale

The presentation summarized here conveys the emergence and value of research on the impact of maltreatment on child and adolescent neurological development and highlights the advantageous perspective of considering differences between maltreated children who are and are not diagnosed with posttraumatic stress disorder (PTSD). Maltreated children are at a particularly high risk for the development of PTSD; though there are contradictory findings of PTSD prevalence in the literature, select studies show that approximately 40–60% of sexually abused children (Dubner & Motta, 1999; McLeer, Deblinger, Henry, & Orvaschel, 1992), 50% of physically abused children (Green, 1985), and 36% of neglected children exposed to domestic violence (De Bellis, Hooper, Spratt, & Woolley, 2009) have PTSD. These prevalence rates are comparable to those of children exposed to warfare and other deleterious life events. While maltreatment is not the only form of childhood trauma (e.g., loss of a parent), it is known to contribute largely to the presence of PTSD in children.

A developmental traumatology model of child maltreatment (De Bellis, 2001) has been proposed to conceptualize the developmental impact of child maltreatment, particularly through the growth and consequences of attachment disorders;

J. Rock (✉) · C. F. Geier
Department of Human Development and Family Studies, The Pennsylvania State University, State College, PA, USA
e-mail: JAR77@psu.edu

J. G. Noll
The Pennsylvania State University, USA

M. D. De Bellis
Department of Psychiatry and Behavioral Sciences, Duke University School of Medicine, Durham, NC, USA

© Springer International Publishing AG, part of Springer Nature 2018
J. G. Noll, I. Shalev (eds.), *The Biology of Early Life Stress*, Child Maltreatment Solutions Network, https://doi.org/10.1007/978-3-319-72589-5_4

internalizing disorders such as separation anxiety and major depression; externalizing disorders such as attention deficit hyperactivity, oppositional defiance, and suicide attempts; and cognitive and learning disorders and poor school performance. The role of PTSD in creating or exacerbating the developmental impact of trauma is consequential and should be the focus of further study. Aside from a societal and ethical obligation to disrupt pathways to negative outcomes for maltreated children, research of this kind is also a matter of resource efficiency in the prevention and reduction of other public health issues such as criminality.

Despite the prevalence rates cited above, scientists and clinicians outside the study and practice of trauma work may make the common mistake of assuming that experiences of trauma and the development of PTSD are one in the same, i.e., that all who have experienced trauma (particularly, severe and/or chronic trauma) must have PTSD. To the contrary, there are important differences between individuals in their response to trauma, and likewise, there exist relevant differences between children in their response to maltreatment. Many maltreated children do not develop PTSD, or if they do, PTSD symptoms subsist after a normative period of time; furthermore, many maltreated children do not go on to have poor commonly associated life experiences, such as academic failure. The pathway from maltreatment to poor life outcomes is not deterministic or inevitable. Considering these differences offers an opportunity to identify compounding developmental factors that may deter maltreated children from the path towards negative outcomes.

4.2 Posttraumatic Stress Disorder Diagnosis

Though many individuals exposed to trauma do not develop a mental health diagnosis, the Diagnostic and Statistical Manual (DSM) IV diagnosis of PTSD does require the experience of a trauma event, which involves actual or threatened injury to the self or others. This event must have resulted in intrusive re-experiencing of trauma (cluster B criterion), which could include having ongoing thoughts and reminders of the trauma experience. As an example, a child whose experience of maltreatment involved loud noises (such as domestic violence) may re-experience his or her trauma when a schoolteacher raises his or her voice. As a result of this triggering experience, the child demonstrates further persistent symptoms. For example, he or she may not be able to concentrate in the school environment and may avoid stimuli and/or demonstrate numbing, emotional bluntedness, and/or dissociation (cluster C criterion). The re-experiencing of trauma may also result in heightened physiological arousal and restlessness (cluster D criterion), such as over-stimulation and fidgeting. This is particularly relevant considering that in comparison with other children, children with PTSD are also more restricted in their expression of emotion. Considering the combination of heightened arousal and restricted self-expression allows us to understand why PTSD is sometimes misdiagnosed, for example, as bipolar disorder or schizophrenia. In order to qualify for the PTSD diagnosis, the duration of symptoms must be greater than 1 month and cause clinically significant distress.

In the most recent update to the Diagnostic and Statistical Manual (DSM-V), the PTSD diagnosis in children is distinguished from the PTSD diagnosis in adults to reflect that younger children (less than 7 years old) may have fewer symptoms than adults but qualify for and be similarly impaired by the disorder. PTSD symptomology is also altered in the DSM-V to include the possible presence of dissociative reactions and flashbacks, the addition of a cluster for numbing of responsiveness and negative beliefs about the world, and the clarification that heightened physiological arousal may include reckless or self-destructive behaviors. The research presented in this summary identifies children with the diagnosis of PTSD who would meet diagnostic criteria in both the DSM-IV and DSM-V.

4.3 Normative Childhood and Adolescent Brain Development

An understanding of the neurobiological impact of trauma requires a foundational consideration of normative childhood and adolescent brain development. Human brain development is marked by the acquisition of progressive skills in cognitive, behavioral, emotional, and physical domains and the complementary neurodevelopmental process of myelination in various regions in which neuronal networks increase connectivity (De Bellis & Zisk, 2014). Popular comparative images of white and gray matter in infant and older child brains reflect the significant growth of neural connections that take place in the early years of childhood, though this neuronal development continues through adolescence and into young adulthood (Giedd & Rapoport, 2010). While some areas of the brain (e.g., the hippocampus) continue to regenerate neurons into adulthood, research substantiates that the first 5 years of life involve significant proliferation of neurons and synaptic connections.

While childhood is a time of unique synaptic changes, the neurological developmental emphasis of adolescence involves the pruning of neural connections and associated "fine tuning" of brain development; as a general rule, the connections that are active and in use are maintained, and the connections that go unused are pruned. These connections are maintained or pruned throughout the brain, including the prefrontal cortex, parietal cortex, temporal lobes, and occipital areas, reaching more adult-like levels of structural maturation at different rates. Overall, these neurobiological growth processes support the development of cognitive skills—including improved memory, problem-solving abilities, mental flexibility, planning, behavioral regulation, and emotional regulation—essential abilities in the response and management of traumatic and stressful life experiences, and those abilities that could also be negatively altered by the experience of trauma and development of PTSD.

4.4 Research on Biological Stress Systems and Adverse Brain Development Mechanisms

Extant research indicates that biological stress systems and inflammatory markers can be dysregulated by early experiences of trauma and that these systemic changes impact further neurological development. This research is reflected in studies on the increases of inflammatory markers and risk for auto-immune disease, catecholamine- and glucocorticoid-induced accelerated loss of neurons (Sapolsky, Uno, Reert, & Finch, 1990; Simantov et al., 1996) resulting in a premature aging process, glucocorticoid-induced delays in myelination (Dunlop, Archer, Quinlivan, Beazley, & Newnham, 1997), glucocorticoid inhibition of neurogenesis (Gould, McEwen, Tanapat, Galea, & Fuchs, 1997; Gould, Tanapat, & Cameron, 1997; Gould, Tanapat, McEwen, Flugge, & Fuchs, 1998), and catecholamine-induced abnormalities in the developmentally appropriate or normative pruning process (Lauder, 1988; Todd, 1992). Neurological scientific studies indicate that the impact of trauma is relevant to development and could have long-lasting consequences.

4.5 Research on Maturation and Cognitive Function in Maltreated Children and Adolescents

Technological progress and increased availability of brain imaging equipment has allowed for new directions in the study of neurological development in maltreated children (among several other important areas of developmental neuroscience). Prior to these advancements, research of this nature on the maltreated child population relied primarily on studies of observed and reported cognitive development (Azar, Barnes, & Twentyman, 1988; Augoustinos, 1987; Beers & De Bellis, 2002; Carrey, Butter, Persingler, & Bialik, 1995; Kolko, 1992; Money, Annecillo, & Kelly, 1983; Perez & Widom, 1994; Trickett, McBride-Chang, & Putnam, 1994), for which only one known study (Perez & Widom, 1994) was longitudinal in nature. Study outcomes largely focused on educational outcomes and indicated that maltreated children were more likely than non-maltreated children to have a lower intelligence quotient and lower academic performance. Without undermining the value of this work, it is widely recognized that there are significant gaps in knowledge about maltreated children's developmental experiences, consequences, limitations, and needs.

In addition to the greater opportunities afforded by brain imaging technology, innovative research has focused on maltreated children who experience health and success in adolescence, for example, young people who are medically healthy despite the presence of traumatic stress (De Bellis & Keshavan, 2003). This perspective has allowed for greater consideration of divergent developmental pathways, appreciation of neurobiological contributions to resilience, and identification of intervention opportunities after child maltreatment (even following experiences that are severe in nature).

4.6 Cortical Region Volume of Maltreated Children and Adolescents

Emerging research on brain maturation and impacted neurocognition in maltreated and/or PTSD-diagnosed children and adolescents substantiates the impact of trauma and stress on neural activity and intracranial volume; while some of these studies consider the overall brain size, others focus on the volume (or lack thereof) in individual cortical regions. Relationships between child maltreatment and brain volume have focused on structures such as the hippocampus, cerebellum, and corpus callosum. In a study of children and adolescents with maltreatment-related PTSD and socio-demographically matched healthy control subjects, anatomical findings from Magnetic Resonance Imaging (MRI) scans indicated that subjects with PTSD, in comparison with healthy controls, had smaller intracranial, cerebral, and prefrontal cortex regions, reduced prefrontal cortical white matter, smaller right temporal lobe volumes, and smaller areas of the corpus callosum and sub-regions, including a smaller midsagittal area of the corpus callosum. In comparison with controls, subjects with PTSD also had proportionally larger right, left, and total lateral ventricles, and a greater amount of cerebrospinal fluid (De Bellis et al., 2002). A commonly used image of the brain of an 11-year-old maltreated male depicts larger lateral ventricles (in comparison to a matched control). Such larger spaces are commonly observed in an aging subject with dementia or severe mental illness, which underlines the severity and concerning relevance of such an observation (Fig. 4.1).

De Bellis and Kuchibhatla (2006) conducted a study of maltreated children and adolescents with PTSD, compared with control groups of children with generalized anxiety disorder (no trauma histories) and healthy adolescents (no trauma histories); cerebellar volumes of maltreated children and adolescents with PTSD (including

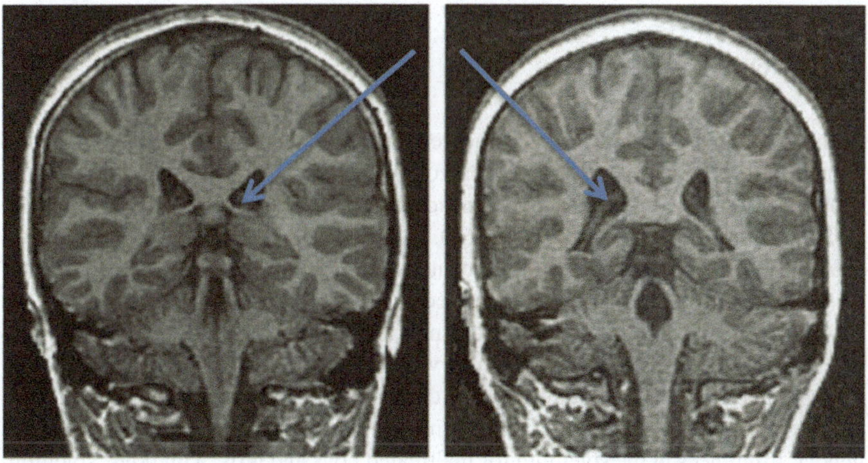

Fig. 4.1 Lateral ventricles in an 11-year-old maltreated male with chronic PTSD (right), compared with a healthy, non-maltreated matched control subject

the left, right, and total cerebellum volume) were significantly smaller. The cerebellum is involved not only in motor movement (the most traditionally recognized functional association), but also increasingly acknowledged for its role in language development, emotional regulation, and reward systems. This region is also known for its significant growth during childhood and adolescence (one of the latest maturing structures, as cited by Giedd and Rapoport 2010) and its relatively low heritability in comparison to other cortical regions (Tiemeier et al., 2010). De Bellis, Keshavan, Clark, et al. (1999) also identified differences between maltreated and non-maltreated children in the corpus callosum, which grows from the interior to the posterior and is also highly involved in attachment and executive functions.

Not all trauma experiences are equal, and as one example of the relevant differences in maltreatment experiences, the *age* at which maltreatment is experienced and the *duration* of the maltreatment experiences appear to play an important role in the neurobiological impact of the trauma. Two studies identified that for maltreated children, brain volumes are positively correlated with the age at onset of maltreatment ($r = 0.40$, $p < 0.05$, De Bellis, Baum, Birmaher, et al., 1999; $r = 0.39$, $p < 0.04$, De Bellis et al., 2002) and negatively correlated with the duration of maltreatment ($r = -0.32$, $p < 0.04$, De Bellis, Baum, Birmaher, et al., 1999; $r = -0.42$, $p < 0.03$, De Bellis et al., 2002). This finding that the earlier a child experiences maltreatment, the smaller their brain size, supports other evidence of the presence of sensitive periods of neurological development. Researchers have also identified a relationship between the years of abuse and intracranial volume in maltreated children with PTSD (De Bellis, Baum, Birmaher, et al., 1999; De Bellis et al., 2002). The aforementioned study of cerebellar volumes (De Bellis & Kuchibhatla, 2006) also substantiates that these volumes are positively correlated with age of onset of trauma leading to PTSD ($r = 0.44$, $p = 0.0005$) and negatively correlated with the duration of trauma ($r = -0.25$, $p = 0.06$).

4.7 Gender Differences

Several studies have indicated that the neurodevelopmental impact for young maltreated males may be greater than for young maltreated females. De Bellis et al. (2002) demonstrated greater lateral ventricle volume increases in male subjects with PTSD than in female subjects with PTSD. De Bellis and Keshavan (2003) compared medically healthy children and adolescents with PTSD to healthy controls, grouped by gender, and found that while all subjects with PTSD had reduced growth in the total corpus callosum compared to non-maltreated subjects, the finding was more prominent in males; furthermore, males with PTSD demonstrated smaller cerebral volumes and rostrum and isthmus areas (corpus callosum regions) in comparison to females with PTSD. De Bellis, Baum, Birmaher, et al. (1999) also found maturational gender differences in the splenium for maltreated boys and girls, with boys' splenium volume more adversely impacted. Other studies have indicated significant gender by PTSD interactions, but there may be no gender differences in the size of the hippocampus or activity of the amygdala for maltreated boys versus maltreated girls. Nonetheless, boys appear to be more vulnerable to developmental trauma disorder.

Prior studies have shown that maltreated males with PTSD show a trend towards more PTSD cluster C symptoms than maltreated females with PTSD; cluster C symptoms represent both avoidant and dissociative behaviors and can be thought of as ways to control painful and distressing re-experiencing of symptoms. Cluster C symptoms can lead to diminished interest in others, feelings of detachment, a restricted range of emotion, and dissociation. Emotional numbing and diminished interest in others, particularly during development, may result in lack of empathy and increased risk for antisocial behaviors. There may be a sociobiological basis to this phenomenon; detachment behaviors during adverse circumstances (such as warfare) would be more beneficial to male than female primitive humans.

4.8 Neurocognitive Function Differences in Maltreated Children With and Without PTSD

A consideration of maltreated children who do not experience adverse brain development has been particularly beneficial to understanding the potentially differing trajectories of maltreated children who do and do not develop PTSD. De Bellis, Woolley, and Hooper (2013) compared maltreated children with PTSD to maltreated children without PTSD and both groups to a control group of healthy, non-maltreated children. This study included children who were previously diagnosed with PTSD but no longer showed signs and symptoms, as well as children who had never been diagnosed despite maltreatment experiences. In order to draw these comparisons, strict clinical inclusion and exclusion methods were utilized. The Kiddie-Sads-Present and Lifetime (K-SADS-PL) assessment for DSM-IV diagnosis of PTSD and other disorders was utilized, and maltreatment was defined and substantiated by child protective services. Included participants lived in a stable home environment, had one non-abusing parent who could cooperate with study protocol, and had access to birth records. Exclusion criteria included participants who used medication with central nervous system effects, had a history of significant medical illness or head injury, experienced obesity or growth failure, had a birth weight under five pounds (or significant prenatal alcohol/drug exposure or birth complications), were diagnosed with anorexia nervosa, autism, pervasive developmental disorder, or schizophrenia, or had a full scale intelligence quotient score of less than 70 for all subjects, or any trauma, maltreatment, or psychiatric illness history for the healthy non-maltreated control subjects.

Interviews with children/adolescents and their parent were conducted in 1 day, including genetic testing of children, cognitive testing of both children and their parents, and mental health interviews of both children and their parents. MRI brain scans for anatomy, Diffusion Tensor Imaging (DTI), Functional Magnetic Resonance Imaging (fMRI), and Magnetic Resonance Spectroscopy (MRS) were completed on separate testing days. Researchers used the Children's Global Assessment Sale (CGAS) and Child Behavior Checklist (CBCL) to document internalizing and externalizing behaviors, as well as measurements of dissociation, total PTSD symptoms, and lifetime summary of maltreatment types, to compare non-maltreated children, maltreated children, and maltreated children with PTSD.

Both maltreated children with PTSD and maltreated children without PTSD performed more poorly than the healthy controls in several areas of cognitive functioning, including intelligence, attention, language, memory, executive functioning, and academic achievement in math and reading. The primary cognitive functioning difference between maltreated children with and without PTSD was on performance of visual-spatial tasks ($F(4, 134) = 4.49$, $p = 0.002$), which has relevance for executive functioning (De Bellis et al., 2013).

In another study grouping maltreated children with PTSD separately from maltreated children without PTSD (and a third group of children without maltreatment experiences), De Bellis et al. (2015) examined anatomical volumetric and corpus callosum DTI measures using MRI scans to find less posterior gray matter volume in children with maltreatment-related PTSD in comparison to maltreated controls. A correlation was identified between total posterior gray matter volumes and the number of PTSD symptoms in maltreated children, such that the greater the number of PTSD symptoms, the lower the posterior gray matter volume ($r = -0.37$, $p < 0.01$). Furthermore, in comparison with the control group, maltreated children without PTSD have a higher volume of cerebellar gray matter, and maltreated children with PTSD have a lower volume of cerebellar gray matter (F2, 113 = 6.7, $p < 0.002$). Similar to the relationship with posterior gray matter, a positive correlation was also found between cerebellum gray matter and PTSD symptoms, such that the greater the number of PTSD symptoms, the smaller the cerebellum ($r = 0.44$, $p < 0.002$). Based on these findings, one might conclude that child maltreatment can lead to "chronic PTSD brain" or "resilience to chronic PTSD brain," differing trajectories that have a substantial impact on the likelihood for further risk.

These findings align with other studies about neurobiological associations of maltreatment-related PTSD, including decreased gray matter, posterior cortex, and cerebellum (including the angular gyrus, cuneus, precuneus, lateral occipital gyrus, superior parietal lobule, posterior cingulate, and visual cortex), and the related functions of visual-spatial processing/decision-making, receptive language, attention and executive functions, the posterior default network, and ventral circuits. Furthermore, gender differences were supported; maltreated males had less gray matter than maltreated females in the left superior prefrontal cortex, a region involved in inhibitory control and risk for impulsivity (De Bellis et al., 2015).

Relevant to these studies is the role of the prefrontal cortex, specifically the ventral medial (or orbital frontal) prefrontal cortex, medial prefrontal (or anterior cingulate) cortex, and the limbic system, including the hippocampus and amygdala. In a third study grouping maltreated children with and without PTSD separately (and including non-maltreated controls), Morey, Haswell, Hooper, and De Bellis (2016) used MRI to demonstrate linear relationships between the ventral medial prefrontal cortex and anterior cingulate cortex volumes; the control group and maltreated children without PTSD were found to have greater volume in these areas than maltreated children with PTSD ($F = 3.6$, $p < 0.03$). Maltreated children without PTSD were also found to have a greater total amygdala volume, particularly larger on the left side, than both maltreated children with PTSD and non-maltreated children ($F = 4.3$, $p < 0.02$). Finally, maltreated children without PTSD were found to have a greater right hippocampal volume than both maltreated children with PTSD and non-maltreated children ($F = 4.2$, $p < 0.02$). These findings have relevance to the consideration of differences in complex functions that may be modulated by stress and impacted by neurotransmitter activity. These findings may also represent a shared trauma mechanism that leads to PTSD, impulsivity (attention deficit hyperactivity disorder), co-morbidity, and poor outcomes.

4.9 Neurobiology of Hope

The consideration of differing neurobiological trajectories from childhood maltreatment presents an opportunity for intervention. After an initial trauma, most individuals have PTSD symptoms that resolve on their own; for example, it is very common for individuals who experience trauma to have high anxiety or trouble sleeping for several days or several weeks, after which the symptoms dissipate. A pathway exists in which otherwise traumatized individuals can learn and grow through a mechanism called "extinction." For example, though a young male who has experienced physical or sexual abuse by an older male may have initial adverse reactions to the presence of other older males, the healthy and non-threatening presence of a safe older male may allow the traumatized young person to restructure his reaction and replace his associations. This type of restructuring or replacement of unhealthy associations may be supported through the use of cognitive behavioral therapy (CBT), a preferred treatment option; in a review of recent fMRI studies, Porto et al. (2009, as cited in De Bellis & Zisk, 2014) demonstrated that CBT can relieve dysregulation of fear response and negative emotions associated with anxiety. A trauma-focused adaptation of the CBT intervention is particularly relevant. It should be noted that the effectiveness of changing cognitive responses to fear requires an intact ventral medial prefrontal cortex that can inhibit a fear response to the amygdala and interior cingulate cortex (the ventral medial prefrontal cortex is also known to have value in adolescence for the prediction of later drug use, a compounding risk factor). The early identification of PTSD symptoms following early childhood trauma can allow opportunities to prevent and intervene in this pathway while neurobiological potential is still present (De Bellis, 2001).

In addition to the individual use of cognitive behavioral therapy, there is increasing emphasis on evidence-based programming for maltreated children at risk for PTSD and associated negative life outcomes in the family system. Emerging research indicates the amenability of child maltreatment to primary prevention, such as the Nurse-Family Partnership Program, in which expectant mothers in low-income, at-risk families are visited by nurses. Several studies of this program indicate improved later outcomes for children, including greater educational achievement in childhood, decreased internalizing symptoms and decreased substance use in childhood, and decreased antisocial behaviors in young adulthood (Olds et al., 2007; Kitzman et al., 2010; Eckenrode et al., 2010, as cited in De Bellis & Zisk, 2014).

Overall, adverse brain development may be reversible. When rescued from extremely neglectful and abusive environments, some profoundly maltreated children are capable of accelerated rates of catch-up growth, including remission of severe psychopathology and normalization of cognitive function. There is even capacity for neurogenesis in the adult human brain, though this can be inhibited by other environmental stressors, which may be probabilistic for high-risk individuals. Though "rescuing" is not always possible, understanding how and why some maltreated children do not develop PTSD or adverse brain developmental effects allows researchers, clinicians, program developers, and policy makers to focus on the what, where, and when of intervention that may deter more maltreated children from further negative life consequences. The presenter concludes with the importance of support for longitudinal imaging studies of maltreated children and studies that begin prior to the birth of at-risk children, towards the identification of neurobiological sources of protection and resilience.

References

Augoustinos, M. (1987). Developmental effects of child abuse: A number of recent findings. *Child Abuse & Neglect, 11*, 15–27.

Azar, S. T., Barnes, K. T., & Twentyman, C. T. (1988). Developmental outcomes in abused children: Consequences of parental abuse or a more general breakdown in caregiver behavior? *Behavior Therapist, 11*, 27–32.

Beers, S., & De Bellis, M. D. (2002). Neuropsychological function in children with maltreatment-related posttraumatic stress disorder. *American Journal of Psychiatry, 159*(3), 483–486.

Carrey, N. J., Butter, H. J., Persingler, M. A., & Bialik, R. J. (1995). Physiological and cognitive correlates of child abuse. *Journal of American Academy of Child and Adolescent Psychiatry, 34*(8), 1067–1075.

De Bellis, M. D. (2001). Developmental traumatology: The psychobiological development of maltreated children and its implications for research, treatment, and policy. *Development and Psychopathology, 13*, 539–564.

De Bellis, M. D., Baum, A. S., Birmaher, B., Keshavan, M. S., Eccard, C. H., Boring, A. M., … Ryan, N. D. (1999). Developmental traumatology part I: Biological stress systems. *Society of Biological Psychiatry, 45*, 1259–1270.

De Bellis, M. D., Hooper, S., Spratt, E. G., & Woolley, D. W. (2009). Neuropsychological findings in childhood neglect and their relationships to pediatric PTSD. *Journal of the International Neuropsychological Society, 15*, 1–11.

De Bellis, M. D., Hooper, S. R., Chen, S. D., Provenzale, J. M., Boyd, B. D., Glessner, C. E., … Woolley, D. P. (2015). Posterior structural volumes differ in maltreated youth with and without posttraumatic stress disorder. *Development and Psychopathology, 27*, 1555–1576.

De Bellis, M. D., & Keshavan, M. S. (2003). Sex differences in brain maturation in maltreatment-related pediatric posttraumatic stress disorder. *Neuroscience and Biobehavioral Reviews, 27*, 103–117.

De Bellis, M. D., Keshavan, M. S., Clark, D. B., Casey, B. J., Giedd, J. N., Boring, A. M., … Ryan, N. D. (1999). Developmental traumatology part II: Brain development. *Society of Biological Psychiatry, 45*, 1271–1284.

De Bellis, M. D., Keshavan, M. S., Shifflett, H., Iyengar, S., Beers, S. R., Hall, J., & Moritz, G. (2002). Brain structures in pediatric maltreatment-related posttraumatic stress disorder: A sociodemographically matched study. *Society of Biological Psychiatry, 52*, 1066–1078.

De Bellis, M. D., & Kuchibhatla, M. (2006). Cerebellar volumes in pediatric maltreatment-related posttraumatic stress disorder. *Society of Biological Psychiatry, 60*, 697–703.

De Bellis, M. D., Woolley, D. P., & Hooper, S. R. (2013). Neuropsychological findings in pediatric maltreatment: Relationship of PTSD, dissociative symptoms, and abuse/neglect indices to neurocognitive outcomes. *Child Maltreatment, 18*(3), 171–183.

De Bellis, M. D., & Zisk, A. B. (2014). The biological effects of childhood trauma. *Child and Adolescent Psychiatric Clinics of North America, 23*(2), 185–222.

Dubner, A. E., & Motta, R. W. (1999). Sexually and physically abused foster care children and posttraumatic stress disorder. *Journal of Consulting & Clinical Psychology, 67*, 367–373.

Dunlop, S. A., Archer, M. A., Quinlivan, J. A., Beazley, L. D., & Newnham, J. P. (1997). Repeated prenatal corticosteroids delay myelination in the ovine central nervous system. *Journal of Maternal-Fetal Medicine, 6*, 309–313.

Eckenrode, J., Campa, M., Luckey, D. W., Henderson, C. R., Cole, R., Kitzman, H., … Olds, D. (2010). Long-term effects of prenatal and infancy nurse home visitation on the life course of youths. *Archives of Pediatrics & Adolescent Medicine, 164*(1), 89–98.

Giedd, J. N., & Rapoport, J. L. (2010). Structural MRI of pediatric brain development: What have we learned and where are we going? *Neuron, 67*(5), 728–734.

Gould, E., McEwen, B. S., Tanapat, P., Galea, L. A., & Fuchs, E. (1997). Neurogeneisis in the dentate gyrus of the adult tree shrew is regulated by psychosocial stress and NMDA receptor activation. *Journal of Neuroscience, 17*, 2492–2498.

Gould, E., Tanapat, P., & Cameron, H. A. (1997). Adrenal steroids suppress granule cell death in the developing dentate gyrus through an NMDA receptor-dependent mechanism. *Developmental Brain Research, 103*, 91–93.

Gould, E., Tanapat, P., McEwen, B. S., Flugge, G., & Fuchs, E. (1998). Proliferation of granule cell precursors in the dentate gyrus of adult monkeys is diminished by stress. *Proceedings of the National Academy of Sciences of the United States of America, 95*, 3168–3171.

Green, A. (1985). *Children traumatized by physical abuse*. Washington, DC: American Psychiatric Press.

Kitzman, H. J., Olds, D. L., Cole, R. E., Hanks, C. A., Anson, E. A., Arcoleo, K. J., … Holmberg, J. R. (2010). Enduring effects of prenatal and infancy home visiting by nurses on children. *Archives of Pediatrics & Adolescent Medicine, 164*(5), 412–418.

Kolko, D. (1992). Characteristics of child victims of physical violence: Research findings and clinical implications. *Journal of Interpersonal Violence, 7*, 244–276.

Lauder, J. M. (1988). Neurotransmitters as morphogens. *Progress in Brain Research, 73*, 365–388.

McLeer, S., Deblinger, E., Henry, D., & Orvaschel, H. (1992). Sexually abused children at high risk for post-traumatic stress disorder. *Journal of Child and Adolescent Psychiatry, 31*, 875–879.

Money, J., Annecillo, C., & Kelly, J. F. (1983). Abuse-dwarfism syndrome: After rescue, statural and intellectual catchup growth correlate. *Journal of Clinical Child Psychology, 12*, 279–283.

Morey, R. A., Haswell, C. C., Hooper, S. R., & De Bellis, M. D. (2016). Amygdala, hippocampus, and ventral medial prefrontal cortex volumes differ in maltreated youth with and without post-traumatic stress disorder. *Neuropsychopharmacology, 41*, 791–801.

Olds, D. L., Kitzman, H., Hanks, C., Cole, R., Anson, E., Sidora-Arcoleo, K., … Bondy, J. (2007). Effects of nurse home visiting on maternal and child functioning: Age-9 follow-up of a randomized trial. *Pediatrics, 120*(4), e832–e845.

Perez, C., & Widom, C. S. (1994). Childhood victimization and long-term intellectual and academic outcomes. *Child Abuse & Neglect, 18*(8), 617–633.

Porto, P. R., Oliveira, L., Mari, J., Volchan, E., Figueira, I., & Ventura, P. (2009). Does cognitive Behavioral therapy change the brain? A systematic review of neuroimaging in anxiety disorders. *The Journal of Neuropsychiatry and Clinical Neurosciences, 21*(2), 114–125.

Sapolsky, R. M., Uno, H., Reert, C. S., & Finch, C. E. (1990). Hippocampal damage associated with prolonged glucocorticoid exposure in primates. *Journal of Neuroscience, 10*, 2897–2902.

Simantov, R., Blinder, E., Ratovitski, T., Tauber, M., Gabbay, M., & Porat, S. (1996). Dopamine induced apoptosis in human neuronal cells: Inhibition by nucleic acids antisense to the dopamine transporter. *Neuroscience, 74*, 39–50.

Tiemeier, H., Lenroot, R., Greenstein, D., Tran, L., Pierson, R., & Giedd, J. N. (2010). Cerebellum development during childhood and adolescence: A longitudinal morphometric MRI study. *NeuroImage, 49*(1), 63–70.

Todd, R. D. (1992). Neural development is regulated by classical neuro-transmitters: Dopamine D2 receptor stimulation enhances neurite outgrowth. *Biological Psychiatry, 31*, 794–807.

Trickett, P. K., McBride-Chang, C., & Putnam, F. W. (1994). The classroom performance and behavior of sexually abused girls. *Development and Psychopathology, 6*, 183–194.

Chapter 5
Childhood Maltreatment and Pediatric PTSD: Abnormalities in Threat Neural Circuitry

Ryan Herringa

5.1 Introduction

Childhood maltreatment is regrettably common, affecting an estimated 1 in 4 youth by the age of 18 (Finkelhor, Turner, Shattuck, & Hamby, 2013). Childhood maltreatment accounts for up to 45% of the risk for childhood-onset psychiatric disorders (Green et al., 2010), making it one of the most identifiable and potent risk factors known for mental illness. On the other hand, many youth show emotional adaptation even in the face of severe maltreatment and do not develop mental illness (Daskalakis, Bagot, Parker, Vinkers, & de Kloet, 2013; DuMont, Widom, & Czaja, 2007). What, then, are the neurobiological pathways that may lead to vulnerability or adaptation following maltreatment? Such knowledge is vital for predicting individual outcomes following maltreatment, determining which youth should receive early intervention, and developing biologically informed treatments for symptomatic youth. Studies in my own lab and others have begun to detail abnormalities in the neural circuitry processing threat and fear responses in relation to childhood maltreatment and PTSD. In this chapter, I will review my laboratory's work using functional brain MRI to explore these relationships across adult and pediatric samples. Here, I propose a model in which maltreatment generally leads to neural changes allowing heightened threat detection, which may serve as an adaptive response for children in a dangerous environment. However, a child or adult's ability to recruit prefrontal regulatory regions may play a key role in determining adaptive and maladaptive emotional outcomes following childhood maltreatment.

R. Herringa (✉)
Department of Psychiatry, University of Wisconsin School of Medicine and Public Health, Madison, WI, USA
e-mail: herringa@wisc.edu

© Springer International Publishing AG, part of Springer Nature 2018

J. G. Noll, I. Shalev (eds.), *The Biology of Early Life Stress*, Child Maltreatment Solutions Network, https://doi.org/10.1007/978-3-319-72589-5_5

5.2 Neural Circuitry Underlying Threat Processing and Developmental Considerations

Studies spanning animal models and humans have identified a canonical set of brain regions involved in the detection, processing, and regulation of threat responses. Perhaps most well known of these is the amygdala, a region involved in the detection of salient cues in the environment such as threat, and which is capable of initiating defensive threat responses in the form of the fight-or-flight response (Hartley & Phelps, 2010). The amygdala does not act in isolation, however, and coordinates with other brain regions to enhance or inhibit threat responses. The hippocampus is one such region that is capable of contextually limiting threat responses in an environment otherwise known to be safe (Maren, Phan, & Liberzon, 2013). The ventromedial prefrontal cortex (vmPFC) is involved in stimulus valuation and can automatically inhibit amygdala-based fear responses, as in fear extinction (Milad & Quirk, 2012). Conversely, the anterior midcingulate cortex (aMCC), broadly involved in behavioral adaptation (Shackman et al., 2011), may augment threat responses consistent with its role in conditioned fear (Milad & Quirk, 2012). Finally, dorsal prefrontal regions such as the dorsomedial and dorsolateral prefrontal cortex (dm/dlPFC) are involved in more conscious or effortful appraisal of threat and are capable of downregulating threat responses through connections with the vmPFC and amygdala (Kalisch & Gerlicher, 2014; Phillips, Ladouceur, & Drevets, 2008).

These brain regions, and the connections between them, are not fully developed at birth and are thus susceptible to the effects of childhood maltreatment. For example, amygdala and hippocampal volumes increase rapidly in children up to age 5 and 10, respectively (Uematsu et al., 2012), while higher-level cognitive regulatory regions such as the dorsal prefrontal cortex do not fully mature until the mid-20s (Giedd et al., 2009). Accordingly, functional MRI studies in youth show decreasing amygdala activation in response to emotional stimuli with age, which appears to be linked to stronger coupling between the amygdala and prefrontal regulatory regions (Gee et al., 2013; Vink, Derks, Hoogendam, Hillegers, & Kahn, 2014). It stands to reason, then, that maltreatment may bias these neurodevelopmental trajectories both in ways that are adaptive for a stressful environment and in other ways that may lead to vulnerability for psychopathology such as anxiety, depression, and PTSD.

5.3 Childhood Maltreatment and Functional Brain Abnormalities

Many neuroimaging studies have documented neural abnormalities during emotion processing in relation to childhood maltreatment and other forms of adversity. For example, amygdala hyperactivation has been reported across many types of childhood adversity (e.g., poverty, caregiver deprivation, interpersonal violence, maltreatment, and stressful life events) (Garrett et al., 2012; Gee et al., 2013; Kim et al.,

2013; McCrory et al., 2011; McLaughlin, Peverill, Gold, Alves, & Sheridan, 2015; Swartz, Williamson, & Hariri, 2015; Dannlowski et al., 2012, 2013; Suzuki et al., 2014; Maheu et al., 2010; Malter Cohen et al., 2013; Tottenham et al., 2011) and appears to be specific to negative emotional stimuli (Dannlowski et al., 2013; Gee, Gabard-Durnam, et al., 2013; Maheu et al., 2010; McLaughlin et al., 2015) [though see (Suzuki et al., 2014)] but is generally independent of symptom levels (Dannlowski et al., 2012, 2013; Garrett et al., 2012; Gee, Gabard-Durnam, et al., 2013; Kim et al., 2013; McCrory et al., 2011; McLaughlin et al., 2015; Suzuki et al., 2014; Swartz et al., 2015). In contrast, prefrontal findings during emotion processing have been more variable and include mixed findings (increased and decreased activation) in the mPFC (Crozier, Wang, Huettel, & De Bellis, 2014; Garrett et al., 2012), dlPFC (Fonzo, Huemer, & Etkin, 2016; Garrett et al., 2012; Kim et al., 2013; McLaughlin et al., 2015), and ventrolateral (vl)PFC (Crozier et al., 2014; Garrett et al., 2012; Gee, Gabard-Durnam, et al., 2013; Kim et al., 2013) in relation to maltreatment. Notably, abnormal prefrontal activation may also be specific to negative stimuli (Gee, Gabard-Durnam, et al., 2013; McLaughlin et al., 2015), further implicating neurodevelopmental abnormalities in threat processing following maltreatment. However, it remains unclear which abnormalities may contribute to adaptive or maladaptive emotional responses following maltreatment and how brain networks, and not just specific brain regions, have been impacted. In the following section, I review studies in my laboratory examining these questions.

5.4 Maltreatment and Resting-State Brain Functional Connectivity

Resting-state fMRI offers a method of probing the brain's intrinsic networks and connectivity in the absence of specific task demands (Fox & Raichle, 2007). As such, it offers a view of brain function that goes beyond a single experimental task design. Using resting-state scans, we examined the relationship between childhood maltreatment and amygdala and hippocampus functional connectivity in a group of 64 late adolescents (age 18) who participated in the longitudinal Wisconsin Study of Families and Work (Herringa et al., 2013). We measured childhood maltreatment by self-report using the Childhood Trauma Questionnaire (CTQ), a well-validated measure of maltreatment experiences (Bernstein et al., 2003). In this study, childhood maltreatment was associated with reduced connectivity between both the amygdala and hippocampus and the vmPFC (Fig. 5.1). Furthermore, maltreatment was associated with a greater reduction in amygdala–vmPFC connectivity in girls compared to boys. Together, these findings suggest that maltreatment may weaken a key circuit involved in the automatic inhibition of threat responses. Presumably, this could occur through weakened inhibitory control of the amygdala by the vmPFC and by impaired ability of the vmPFC to contextually limit threat responses via information derived from the hippocampus. Reduced amygdala– and

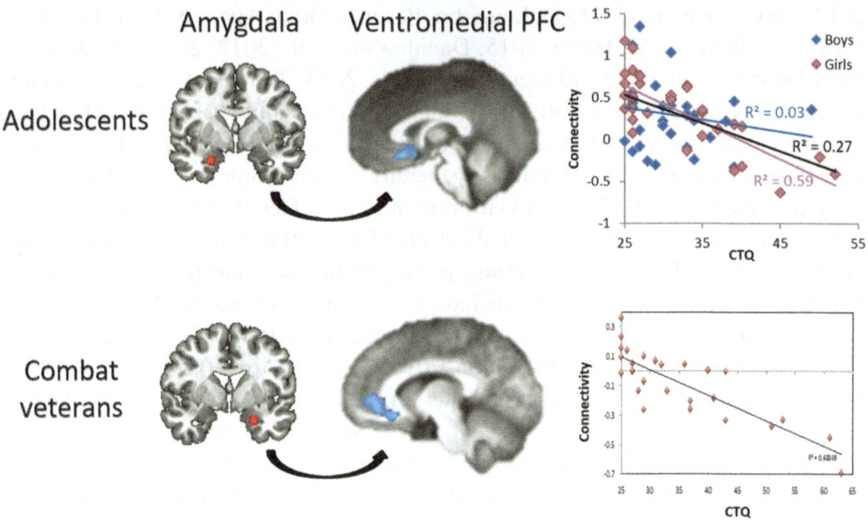

Fig. 5.1 Childhood maltreatment is associated with reduced resting-state connectivity between the amygdala and ventromedial prefrontal cortex (PFC). This effect was present in a community sample of adolescents (top) and in young adult combat veterans (bottom). *CTQ* Childhood Trauma Questionnaire. Figure adapted from Birn et al. (2014) and Herringa, Phillips, et al. (2013)

hippocampus–vmPFC connectivity also partially mediated internalizing symptoms of anxiety and depression at age 18, suggesting that maltreatment-related abnormalities in these circuits confer some risk for psychiatric problems.

In another study, we examined the relationship between childhood maltreatment and amygdala and hippocampus resting-state connectivity in a sample of young adult combat veterans from the Iraq and Afghanistan wars (ave. 26.6 years) (Birn, Patriat, Phillips, Germain, & Herringa, 2014). Within this analysis, we also examined the unique relationships of combat exposure and combat PTSD symptoms to amygdala and hippocampal connectivity, allowing us to differentiate between the effects of childhood and adult trauma as well as symptom levels. Similar to the adolescent study, we found that childhood maltreatment was associated with reduced connectivity between the amygdala and hippocampus and the vmPFC (Fig. 5.1). However, childhood maltreatment was also associated with greater coupling (more anticorrelation) between the amygdala/hippocampus and dmPFC (Fig. 5.2), a region involved in the cognitive control of emotion, as noted above. Furthermore, PTSD symptoms were associated with reduced coupling (less anticorrelation) between the amygdala/hippocampus and dm/dlPFC (Fig. 5.2). These results suggest that maltreatment may weaken ventral automatic regulatory circuits that inhibit threat responses, but which may be largely adaptive in allowing for enhanced threat detection and initial response. However, maltreatment may also augment coupling with dorsal prefrontal regions involved in the effortful, cognitive control of threat. Conversely, PTSD symptoms may emerge from a weakening of

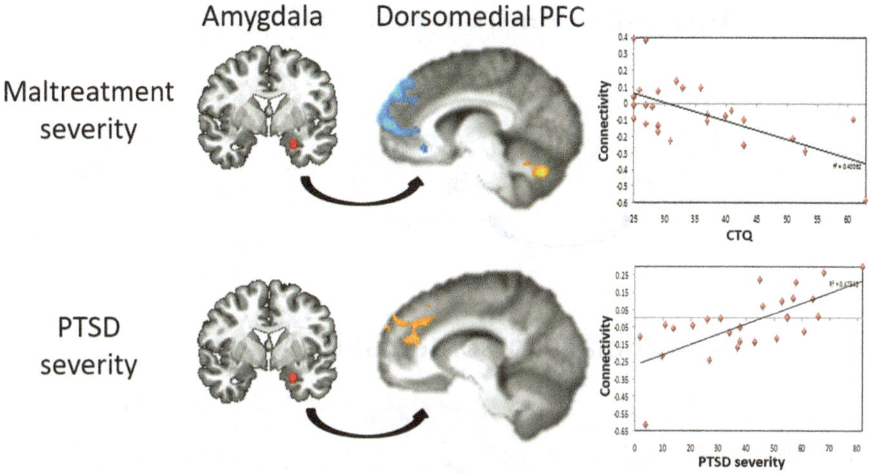

Fig. 5.2 Combat veterans show differential effects of childhood maltreatment and combat PTSD on amygdala-dorsomedial prefrontal cortex (dmPFC) resting-state connectivity. Childhood maltreatment is associated with greater negative coupling (anticorrelation) between the amygdala and dmPFC (top). However, combat PTSD symptoms are associated with a loss of this anticorrelation. Negative coupling between the amygdala and dmPFC is typical of healthy adults. Figure adapted from Birn et al. (2014)

cognitive control connections, suggesting a potential pathway by which cumulative trauma may lead to psychopathology.

5.5 Maltreatment and Brain Functional Connectivity During Emotion Processing

The above studies suggest maltreatment-related abnormalities in the resting state function of threat circuits. Are similar abnormalities present during emotion processing, and do we see evidence of abnormal neurodevelopment in affected youth? To answer these questions, we conducted a functional MRI study in a sample of approximately 30 youth with PTSD and 30 healthy youth between the ages of 8 and 18 years (ave. 14 years). Index traumas for the PTSD group consisted primarily of interpersonal violence, including abuse. Youth performed two emotion-processing tasks, in which they viewed standardized neutral and threat scenes, and a task viewing emotional faces (angry, happy). The groups were similar in terms of age, IQ, and pubertal status.

In the analysis of threat vs. neutral scenes (Wolf & Herringa, 2016), there were surprisingly no differences in amygdala activation between the two groups. However, youth with PTSD showed hyperactivation in the aMCC, a region notable for its role in enhancing conditioned threat responses. Furthermore, while youth with PTSD did not show differential amygdala activation, they did have weaker

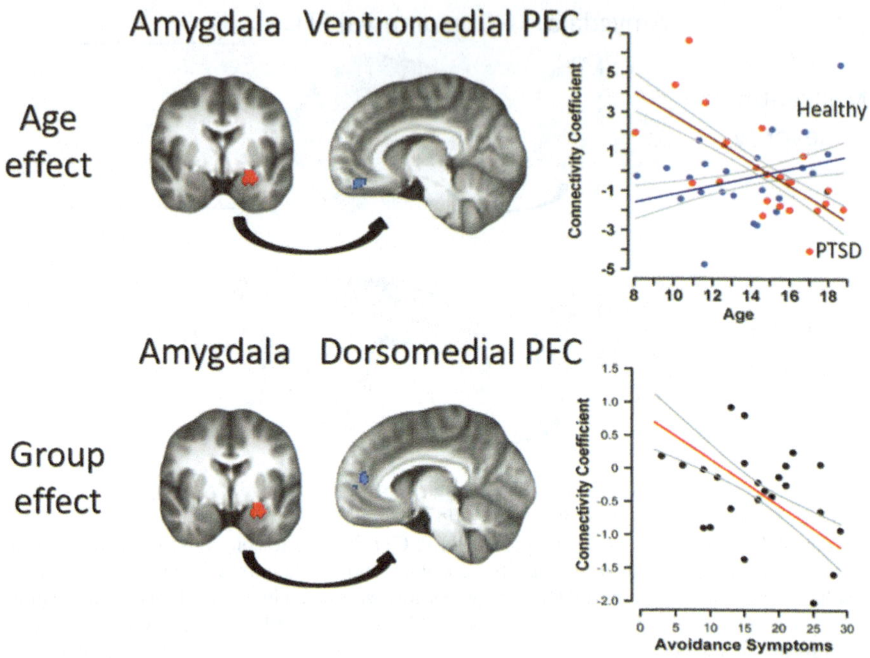

Fig. 5.3 Functional brain abnormalities during viewing of threat vs. neutral scenes in youth with PTSD. Youth with PTSD show age-related differences in amygdala-ventromedial prefrontal cortex connectivity (top). Here, youth with PTSD show decreased coupling with age, the opposite pattern of healthy youth. Youth with PTSD also show reduced coupling between the amygdala and dorsomedial prefrontal cortex (PFC) when viewing threat scenes, which was also associated with greater PTSD avoidance symptoms (bottom). Figure adapted from Wolf and Herringa (2016)

coupling between the amygdala and dmPFC, which also related to PTSD severity (Fig. 5.3). Additionally, this analysis revealed age-related differences in functional connectivity between the amygdala and vmPFC. Here, healthy youth showed increasing connectivity with age, while youth with PTSD showed decreasing connectivity (Fig. 5.3). Notably, amygdala-vmPFC connectivity was not associated with PTSD severity. These findings agree overall with an emerging model suggested by the resting-state studies, in which maltreatment experiences may weaken more automatic ventral regulatory circuits over the course of development but may also confer adaptive benefit in a dangerous environment. However, weakened coupling between the amygdala and dorsal cognitive control regions may underlie (at least in part) the expression of PTSD in youth.

In the emotional faces task, we examined brain activation and amygdala functional connectivity for happy and angry faces compared to a shape control condition (Keding & Herringa, 2016). While we again detected no overall differences in amygdala activation, we did observe a developmental effect. Healthy youth showed decreasing amygdala activation to emotional faces with age, consistent with prior work in normative samples of youth. However, youth with PTSD showed increasing

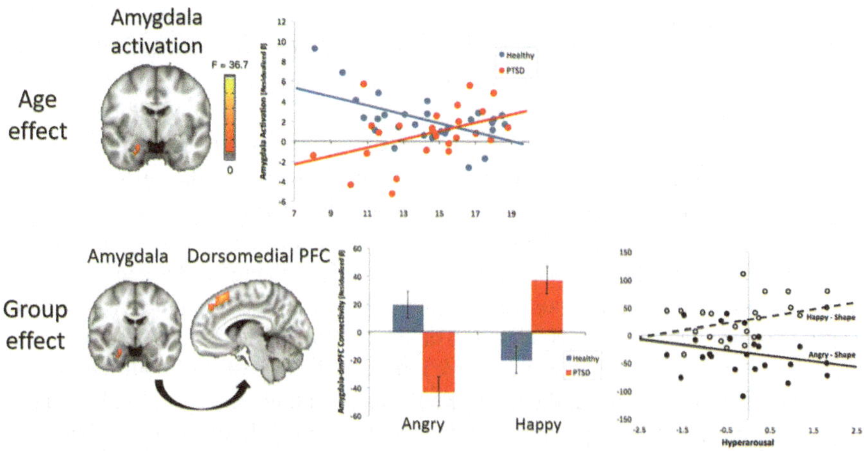

Fig. 5.4 Functional brain abnormalities during viewing of emotional faces in youth with PTSD. Youth with PTSD show age-related differences in amygdala activation (top). Here, youth with PTSD show increased activation with age, the opposite pattern of healthy youth. Youth with PTSD also show reduced coupling between the amygdala and dorsomedial prefrontal cortex (PFC) when viewing angry faces but increased coupling when viewing happy faces (bottom). This emotion-abnormal connectivity was further associated with PTSD hyperarousal symptoms. Figure adapted from Keding and Herringa (2016)

amygdala activation with age, which was unrelated to symptom severity (Fig. 5.4). When examining aMCC activation, we found, somewhat to our surprise, that youth with PTSD showed no differential activation to angry faces but did show hyperactivation to happy faces. Furthermore, we observed a similar interaction in amygdala–dmPFC connectivity. Here, youth with PTSD showed decreased connectivity to angry faces but increased amygdala-dmPFC connectivity to happy faces (Fig. 5.4). These emotion-specific abnormalities were further linked to PTSD severity, suggesting they represent a maladaptive response to maltreatment. Specifically, pediatric PTSD appears to be associated with insufficient deployment of appraisal and regulatory resources to typical threat (angry faces) but excessive resource deployment to typically safe stimuli (happy faces). Consistent with our other work, these findings also suggest that dysfunction in a key cognitive-emotional control circuit (amygdala to dorsal prefrontal cortex) may play a key role in determining adaptive and maladaptive emotional responses following maltreatment.

5.6 A Model of Adaptive and Maladaptive Changes in Threat Circuitry Following Maltreatment

What do these findings tell us about how childhood maltreatment impacts the developing brain's threat circuitry? Which neural "changes" may confer adaptive benefits for youth, and which may contribute to psychiatric illness? These are ultimately very difficult questions to answer for several reasons. First, we do not have a clear measure of how certain biological or behavioral changes may have allowed a child to adapt to her environment. Do we measure academic success, intensity or frequency of emotion, or ability to avoid future danger? Second, any "adaptive" brain changes that allow a child to survive in an abusive environment, and at a certain age, could become maladaptive in other circumstances. Hypervigilance to emotional faces could be helpful while living with an abusive caregiver but could become problematic in forming peer relationships, moving to a safe household, or seeking a job as an adult. In other words, while the *context* has changed, the neural systems remain primed for a dangerous environment. Third, we do not know whether the observed neural abnormalities related to maltreatment were present before maltreatment occurred (i.e., a predisposing factor), occurred as a result of maltreatment, or were due to another confounding factor such as pollutant exposure, food availability, or intrauterine drug exposure. Finally, fMRI is limited in its ability to determine actual function at the neuronal circuit level. For example, does a greater fMRI signal in the amygdala signify activation of inhibitory neurons, excitatory neurons, or both, and in which subnuclei of the amygdala? The implications of activation findings can be drastically different depending on the answers to such questions. Clearly, we must remain humble in interpreting human neuroimaging studies such as these and seek to either support or refute these findings with longitudinal studies in humans and animal models.

With the above caveats noted, I will propose a model of adaptive and maladaptive neural changes following maltreatment that can offer testable hypotheses in future work (Fig. 5.5). As an admittedly coarse measure, I will use clinical symptom relationships as a barometer of emotional adaptation. In other words, abnormalities clearly linked to anxiety, depression, or PTSD severity are seen as more likely to represent maladaptive neural function caused by maltreatment. Using this framework, our findings suggest a number of maltreatment-related brain findings that are likely to be adaptive. These findings include increasing amygdala activation with age, weaker coupling with age between the amygdala/hippocampus and vmPFC, and aMCC hyperactivation to canonical threats. Together, these network changes may allow for heightened automatic detection of threat and appraisal of potential threat. Here, the amygdala can more readily detect potentially salient and threatening cues in the environment, such as an emotional expression, but with less "automatic braking" applied by the vmPFC and hippocampus. This information can then be passed on to the aMCC, which is involved in automatic appraisal processes (deciding whether something is a threat or not). These neural changes could serve to protect a child in an abusive environment so long as potential threat is accurately categorized at the automatic, subconscious level. Our findings in the aMCC are all the more interesting in this regard. Youth with PTSD showed aMCC hyperactivation to threat scenes that was not associated with symptom severity and bears resemblance to normative changes seen in the aMCC in combat veterans (Herringa, Phillips, Fournier, Kronhaus, & Germain, 2013; van Wingen, Geuze, Vermetten, & Fernandez, 2011). On the other hand, youth with PTSD also showed aMCC hyperactivation to happy, but not angry, emotional faces, which was further linked to

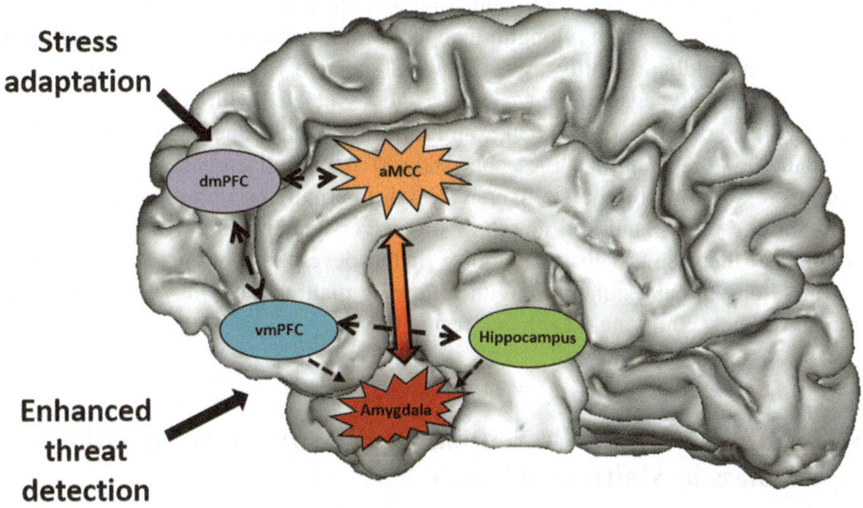

Fig. 5.5 Neural model of adaptive and maladaptive effects of maltreatment on brain function in youth. Maltreatment may elicit hyperactivation in brain regions such as the amygdala and anterior midcingulate cortex (aMCC) which could allow for enhanced automatic detection and appraisal of threat. Emotional adaptation may be determined, however, by the degree of recruitment in cognitive control regions such as the dorsomedial prefrontal cortex (dmPFC), which is involved in the conscious appraisal of threat and emotion regulation. *vmPFC* ventromedial prefrontal cortex

illness severity. This finding would suggest that automatic appraisal of threat for emotional faces may be inappropriately encoded in the aMCC in youth with PTSD and may contribute to difficulties discriminating threat and safety in others' emotional expressions.

Our findings also implicate coupling between the amygdala and dm/dlPFC as being a key determinant of emotional adaptation following maltreatment. In this model, heightened sensitivity of a "bottom-up" threat detection system is balanced by increased engagement of "top-down" control by regulatory prefrontal regions. The dmPFC fits nicely in this regard, as it has been implicated in effortful, conscious threat appraisal (Kalisch & Gerlicher, 2014), can augment or inhibit threat responses based on context (Robinson, Charney, Overstreet, Vytal, & Grillon, 2012), and is associated with emotion regulation success and lower anxiety via coupling with the amygdala (Kim, Gee, Loucks, Davis, & Whalen, 2011; Lee, Heller, van Reekum, Nelson, & Davidson, 2012). The adaptive upregulation of dm/dlPFC following maltreatment is also supported by additional recent studies, including our own (Fonzo et al., 2016; Herringa et al., 2016; Kim et al., 2013; McLaughlin et al., 2015). For example, McLaughlin and colleagues showed that, controlling for symptom levels, maltreated youth show amygdala hyperactivation when viewing, but not when regulating emotional reaction to, negative pictures (McLaughlin et al., 2015). Furthermore, maltreated youth showed heightened dm/dlPFC recruitment during emotion regulation, suggesting this is a compensatory mechanism that may support conscious appraisal and emotion regulation. Recent work from our own group also supports this view. In our longitudinal community sample of adolescents, we showed that childhood family adversity was associated with amygdala hyperactivation in response to negative images but was not associated with internalizing symptoms (Herringa et al., 2016). When examining amygdala connectivity, however, low internalizing ("resilient") adolescents showed increased amygdala-dmPFC coupling in relation to childhood adversity. High internalizing ("vulnerable") adolescents, on the other hand, did not show this adversity-related enhancement. These findings further suggest that the ability of the developing brain to augment this cognitive-emotional regulatory circuit following maltreatment may be a key determinant of one's emotional health and resilience.

5.7 Implications for Prevention and Treatment of Mental Illness in Maltreated Youth

I end this chapter by considering the potential implications of these neuroimaging studies for clinicians, schools, child welfare agencies, and policy makers who have an impact on child development. In an ideal world, we would prevent maltreatment from happening in the first place. While beyond the scope of this chapter, there are emerging programs and policies that seek to do just that, for example through parent training and household economic strengthening (Hillis et al., 2016; Prinz, Sanders, Shapiro, Whitaker, & Lutzker, 2009). Even the best programs and policies, however, are unlikely to prevent all cases of child maltreatment, which behooves us to advance secondary prevention and treatment strategies for these youth. The findings summarized in this chapter suggest that maltreatment causes a cascade of neurobiological changes that could have either adaptive or maladaptive effects in terms of emotional well-being. Notably, hyperactivation of regions such as the amygdala, involved in automatic detection of threat, may be advantageous in a dangerous environment. In this sense, we may expect some degree of threat reactivity to persist in affected youth and can help to normalize these reactions for children and families.

On the other hand, our neural findings suggest that augmenting circuitry involved in the conscious appraisal of threat and regulation of emotion may be helpful. In youth who have been maltreated but have not yet developed psychiatric illness, one could envision secondary prevention strategies that seek to enhance threat discrimination and emotion regulation such as cognitive-behavioral therapy, mindfulness training, and safety planning to avoid future dangerous situations. As our biological markers advance, we may one day be able to target such prevention strategies more precisely, focusing on youth who do not show compensatory or adaptive brain changes. For youth who develop a mental illness such as PTSD, therapeutic strategies such as trauma-focused cognitive behavioral therapy and eye-movement desensitization and reprocessing have already shown effectiveness (Cohen & Mannarino, 2015; Diehle, Opmeer, Boer, Mannarino, & Lindauer, 2014). However, future studies would be helpful to determine how these therapies affect the neural systems of threat and whether this translates to more accurate threat discrimination and improved emotion regulation. Notably, our findings suggest that youth with PTSD may show specific impairments in threat appraisal of emotional faces. Here, the brain appears to "dismiss" potential threats that may seem obvious to emotionally healthy individuals (angry faces), and instead recruits additional threat appraisal resources for typically benign expressions (happy faces). Such findings suggest that helping clinically affected youth to more accurately differentiate emotional expressions in their (safe) caregivers and others may help to make their world more predictable. As with secondary preventions, improvements in biomarkers of maltreatment exposure and PTSD in youth may help to guide such therapies in the future by indicating which youth respond to a particular treatment modality and enabling the use of other modalities or novel treatments for those who do not.

For policy makers, the neurobiological findings summarized here should also impart a degree of urgency and motivation to improve interventions at all levels, from prevention of maltreatment to better clinical treatment. Maltreatment appears to change the structure and function of the developing brain in ways that can be quite harmful, placing the brain on a developmental path that leads to a host of negative physical and mental health outcomes. These injuries are not so obvious as a bruise or a broken bone but are nonetheless present. On the other hand, the developing brain can be quite resilient, allowing a child to recover and thrive if given the right support.

Acknowledgments This work was supported by the American Academy of Child and Adolescent Psychiatry, the Brain and Behavior Research Foundation, the University of Wisconsin School of Medicine and Institute for Clinical and Translational Research, and the National Institute of Mental Health. I am grateful for these sources of support, and for all of the staff, trainees, and participating families who have made this work possible.

References

Bernstein, D. P., Stein, J. A., Newcomb, M. D., Walker, E., Pogge, D., Ahluvalia, T., … Zule, W. (2003). Development and validation of a brief screening version of the Childhood Trauma Questionnaire. *Child Abuse & Neglect, 27*(2), 169–190.

Birn, R. M., Patriat, R., Phillips, M. L., Germain, A., & Herringa, R. J. (2014). Childhood maltreatment and combat posttraumatic stress differentially predict fear-related fronto-subcortical connectivity. *Depression and Anxiety, 31*(10), 880–892. https://doi.org/10.1002/da.22291

Cohen, J. A., & Mannarino, A. P. (2015). Trauma-focused cognitive behavior therapy for traumatized children and families. *Child and Adolescent Psychiatric Clinics of North America, 24*(3), 557–570. https://doi.org/10.1016/j.chc.2015.02.005

Crozier, J. C., Wang, L., Huettel, S. A., & De Bellis, M. D. (2014). Neural correlates of cognitive and affective processing in maltreated youth with posttraumatic stress symptoms: Does gender matter? *Development and Psychopathology, 26*(2), 491–513. https://doi.org/10.1017/S095457941400008X

Dannlowski, U., Kugel, H., Huber, F., Stuhrmann, A., Redlich, R., Grotegerd, D., … Suslow, T. (2013). Childhood maltreatment is associated with an automatic negative emotion processing bias in the amygdala. *Human Brain Mapping, 34*(11), 2899–2909. https://doi.org/10.1002/hbm.22112

Dannlowski, U., Stuhrmann, A., Beutelmann, V., Zwanzger, P., Lenzen, T., Grotegerd, D., … Kugel, H. (2012). Limbic scars: Long-term consequences of childhood maltreatment revealed by functional and structural magnetic resonance imaging. *Biological Psychiatry, 71*(4), 286–293. https://doi.org/10.1016/j.biopsych.2011.10.021

Daskalakis, N. P., Bagot, R. C., Parker, K. J., Vinkers, C. H., & de Kloet, E. R. (2013). The three-hit concept of vulnerability and resilience: Toward understanding adaptation to early-life adversity outcome. *Psychoneuroendocrinology, 38*(9), 1858–1873. https://doi.org/10.1016/j.psyneuen.2013.06.008

Diehle, J., Opmeer, B. C., Boer, F., Mannarino, A. P., & Lindauer, R. J. L. (2014). Trauma-focused cognitive behavioral therapy or eye movement desensitization and reprocessing: What works in children with posttraumatic stress symptoms? A randomized controlled trial. *European Child & Adolescent Psychiatry, 24*(2), 227–236. https://doi.org/10.1007/s00787-014-0572-5

DuMont, K. A., Widom, C. S., & Czaja, S. J. (2007). Predictors of resilience in abused and neglected children grown-up: The role of individual and neighborhood characteristics. *Child Abuse & Neglect, 31*(3), 255–274. https://doi.org/10.1016/j.chiabu.2005.11.015

Finkelhor, D., Turner, H. A., Shattuck, A., & Hamby, S. L. (2013). Violence, crime, and abuse exposure in a national sample of children and youth: An update. *JAMA Pediatrics, 167*(7), 614–621. https://doi.org/10.1001/jamapediatrics.2013.42

Fonzo, G. A., Huemer, J., & Etkin, A. (2016). History of childhood maltreatment augments dorsolateral prefrontal processing of emotional valence in PTSD. *Journal of Psychiatric Research, 74*, 45–54. https://doi.org/10.1016/j.jpsychires.2015.12.015

Fox, M. D., & Raichle, M. E. (2007). Spontaneous fluctuations in brain activity observed with functional magnetic resonance imaging. *Nature Reviews Neuroscience, 8*(9), 700–711. https://doi.org/10.1038/nrn2201

Garrett, A. S., Carrion, V., Kletter, H., Karchemskiy, A., Weems, C. F., & Reiss, A. (2012). Brain activation to facial expressions in youth with PTSD symptoms. *Depression and Anxiety, 29*(5), 449–459. https://doi.org/10.1002/da.21892

Gee, D. G., Gabard-Durnam, L. J., Flannery, J., Goff, B., Humphreys, K. L., Telzer, E. H., … Tottenham, N. (2013). Early developmental emergence of human amygdala-prefrontal connectivity after maternal deprivation. *Proceedings of the National Academy of Sciences of the United States of America, 110*(39), 15638–15643. https://doi.org/10.1073/pnas.1307893110

Gee, D. G., Humphreys, K. L., Flannery, J., Goff, B., Telzer, E. H., Shapiro, M., … Tottenham, N. (2013). A developmental shift from positive to negative connectivity in human amygdala-prefrontal circuitry. *The Journal of Neuroscience, 33*(10), 4584–4593. https://doi.org/10.1523/JNEUROSCI.3446-12.2013

Giedd, J. N., Lalonde, F. M., Celano, M. J., White, S. L., Wallace, G. L., Lee, N. R., & Lenroot, R. K. (2009). Anatomical brain magnetic resonance imaging of typically developing children and adolescents. *Journal of the American Academy of Child and Adolescent Psychiatry, 48*(5), 465–470.

Green, J. G., McLaughlin, K. A., Berglund, P. A., Gruber, M. J., Sampson, N. A., Zaslavsky, A. M., & Kessler, R. C. (2010). Childhood adversities and adult psychiatric disorders in the national comorbidity survey replication I: Associations with first onset of DSM-IV disorders. *Archives of General Psychiatry, 67*(2), 113–123. https://doi.org/10.1001/archgenpsychiatry.2009.186

Hartley, C. A., & Phelps, E. A. (2010). Changing fear: The neurocircuitry of emotion regulation. *Neuropsychopharmacology, 35*(1), 136–146. https://doi.org/10.1038/npp.2009.121

Herringa, R. J., Birn, R. M., Ruttle, P. L., Burghy, C. A., Stodola, D. E., Davidson, R. J., & Essex, M. J. (2013). Childhood maltreatment is associated with altered fear circuitry and increased internalizing symptoms by late adolescence. *Proceedings of the National Academy of Sciences of the United States of America, 110*(47), 19119–19124. https://doi.org/10.1073/pnas.1310766110

Herringa, R. J., Burghy, C. A., Stodola, D. E., Fox, M. E., Davidson, R. J., & Essex, M. J. (2016). Enhanced prefrontal-amygdala connectivity following childhood adversity as a protective mechanism against internalizing in adolescence. *Biological Psychiatry: Cognitive Neuroscience and Neuroimaging, 1*(4), 326–334. https://doi.org/10.1016/j.bpsc.2016.03.003

Herringa, R. J., Phillips, M. L., Fournier, J. C., Kronhaus, D. M., & Germain, A. (2013). Childhood and adult trauma both correlate with dorsal anterior cingulate activation to threat in combat veterans. *Psychological Medicine, 43*(7), 1533–1542. https://doi.org/10.1017/S0033291712002310

Hillis, S., Mercy, J., Saul, J., Gleckel, J., Abad, N., & Kress, H. (2016). THRIVES: Using the best evidence to prevent violence against children. *Journal of Public Health Policy, 37*(Suppl 1), 51–65. https://doi.org/10.1057/s41271-016-0003-6

Kalisch, R., & Gerlicher, A. M. V. (2014). Making a mountain out of a molehill: On the role of the rostral dorsal anterior cingulate and dorsomedial prefrontal cortex in conscious threat appraisal, catastrophizing, and worrying. *Neuroscience & Biobehavioral Reviews, 42*, 1–8. https://doi.org/10.1016/j.neubiorev.2014.02.002

Keding, T. J., & Herringa, R. J. (2016). Paradoxical prefrontal-amygdala recruitment to angry and happy expressions in pediatric posttraumatic stress disorder. *Neuropsychopharmacology, 41*(12), 2903–2912. https://doi.org/10.1038/npp.2016.104

Kim, M. J., Gee, D. G., Loucks, R. A., Davis, F. C., & Whalen, P. J. (2011). Anxiety dissociates dorsal and ventral medial prefrontal cortex functional connectivity with the amygdala at rest. *Cerebral Cortex (New York, N.Y.: 1991), 21*(7), 1667–1673. https://doi.org/10.1093/cercor/bhq237

Kim, P., Evans, G. W., Angstadt, M., Ho, S. S., Sripada, C. S., Swain, J. E., ... Phan, K. L. (2013). Effects of childhood poverty and chronic stress on emotion regulatory brain function in adulthood. *Proceedings of the National Academy of Sciences of the United States of America, 110*(46), 18442–18447. https://doi.org/10.1073/pnas.1308240110

Lee, H., Heller, A. S., van Reekum, C. M., Nelson, B., & Davidson, R. J. (2012). Amygdala-prefrontal coupling underlies individual differences in emotion regulation. *NeuroImage, 62*(3), 1575–1581. https://doi.org/10.1016/j.neuroimage.2012.05.044

Maheu, F. S., Dozier, M., Guyer, A. E., Mandell, D., Peloso, E., Poeth, K., ... Ernst, M. (2010). A preliminary study of medial temporal lobe function in youths with a history of caregiver deprivation and emotional neglect. *Cognitive, Affective & Behavioral Neuroscience, 10*(1), 34–49. https://doi.org/10.3758/CABN.10.1.34

Malter Cohen, M., Jing, D., Yang, R. R., Tottenham, N., Lee, F. S., & Casey, B. J. (2013). Early-life stress has persistent effects on amygdala function and development in mice and humans. *Proceedings of the National Academy of Sciences of the United States of America, 110*(45), 18274–18278. https://doi.org/10.1073/pnas.1310163110

Maren, S., Phan, K. L., & Liberzon, I. (2013). The contextual brain: Implications for fear conditioning, extinction and psychopathology. *Nature Reviews. Neuroscience, 14*(6), 417–428. https://doi.org/10.1038/nrn3492

McCrory, E. J., De Brito, S. A., Sebastian, C. L., Mechelli, A., Bird, G., Kelly, P. A., & Viding, E. (2011). Heightened neural reactivity to threat in child victims of family violence. *Current Biology, 21*(23), R947–R948. https://doi.org/10.1016/j.cub.2011.10.015

McLaughlin, K. A., Peverill, M., Gold, A. L., Alves, S., & Sheridan, M. A. (2015). Child maltreatment and neural systems underlying emotion regulation. *Journal of the American Academy of Child and Adolescent Psychiatry, 54*(9), 753–762. https://doi.org/10.1016/j.jaac.2015.06.010

Milad, M. R., & Quirk, G. J. (2012). Fear extinction as a model for translational neuroscience: Ten years of progress. *Annual Review of Psychology, 63*, 129–151. https://doi.org/10.1146/annurev.psych.121208.131631

Phillips, M. L., Ladouceur, C. D., & Drevets, W. C. (2008). A neural model of voluntary and automatic emotion regulation: implications for understanding the pathophysiology and neurodevelopment of bipolar disorder. *Molecular Psychiatry, 13*(9), 829–857.

Prinz, R. J., Sanders, M. R., Shapiro, C. J., Whitaker, D. J., & Lutzker, J. R. (2009). Population-based prevention of child maltreatment: The U.S. triple P system population trial. *Prevention Science, 10*(1), 1–12. https://doi.org/10.1007/s11121-009-0123-3

Robinson, O. J., Charney, D. R., Overstreet, C., Vytal, K., & Grillon, C. (2012). The adaptive threat bias in anxiety: Amygdala-dorsomedial prefrontal cortex coupling and aversive amplification. *NeuroImage, 60*(1), 523–529. https://doi.org/10.1016/j.neuroimage.2011.11.096

Shackman, A. J., Salomons, T. V., Slagter, H. A., Fox, A. S., Winter, J. J., & Davidson, R. J. (2011). The integration of negative affect, pain and cognitive control in the cingulate cortex. *Nature Reviews. Neuroscience, 12*(3), 154–167. https://doi.org/10.1038/nrn2994

Suzuki, H., Luby, J. L., Botteron, K. N., Dietrich, R., McAvoy, M. P., & Barch, D. M. (2014). Early life stress and trauma and enhanced limbic activation to emotionally valenced faces in depressed and healthy children. *Journal of the American Academy of Child and Adolescent Psychiatry, 53*(7), 800–813.e10. https://doi.org/10.1016/j.jaac.2014.04.013

Swartz, J. R., Williamson, D. E., & Hariri, A. R. (2015). Developmental change in amygdala reactivity during adolescence: Effects of family history of depression and stressful life events. *The American Journal of Psychiatry, 172*(3), 276–283. https://doi.org/10.1176/appi.ajp.2014.14020195

Tottenham, N., Hare, T. A., Millner, A., Gilhooly, T., Zevin, J. D., & Casey, B. J. (2011). Elevated amygdala response to faces following early deprivation. *Developmental Science, 14*(2), 190–204. https://doi.org/10.1111/j.1467-7687.2010.00971.x

Uematsu, A., Matsui, M., Tanaka, C., Takahashi, T., Noguchi, K., Suzuki, M., & Nishijo, H. (2012). Developmental trajectories of amygdala and hippocampus from infancy to early adulthood in healthy individuals. *PLoS One, 7*(10), e46970. https://doi.org/10.1371/journal.pone.0046970

van Wingen, G. A., Geuze, E., Vermetten, E., & Fernandez, G. (2011). The neural consequences of combat stress: Long-term follow-up. *Molecular Psychiatry, 17*(2), 116–118. https://doi.org/10.1038/mp.2011.110

Vink, M., Derks, J. M., Hoogendam, J. M., Hillegers, M., & Kahn, R. S. (2014). Functional differences in emotion processing during adolescence and early adulthood. *NeuroImage, 91*, 70–76. https://doi.org/10.1016/j.neuroimage.2014.01.035

Wolf, R. C., & Herringa, R. J. (2016). Prefrontal-amygdala dysregulation to threat in pediatric post-traumatic stress disorder. *Neuropsychopharmacology, 41*(3), 822–831. https://doi.org/10.1038/npp.2015.209

Chapter 6
Pediatric Posttraumatic Stress

Olivia Altamirano and Victor G. Carrión

Preface Children who experience trauma are at a disadvantage in terms of being able to cope with it; thus their ability to succeed is hindered if they are not offered appropriate resources. Traumatic experiences may include natural catastrophes and physical abuse. Children may also be exposed to adversities including poverty and community violence, which are often chronic difficulties. These stressors can be difficult for a child to manage, especially because children's coping skills are few and not yet well developed. For these reasons, it is important to address stress in children. We must conduct research aimed at understanding their brain development, for example, by investigating biological markers and sociocultural factors influencing growth. Research findings will better inform appropriate diagnosis, if present, and focused treatment when needed. It is imperative to intervene early with children in order to help them gain the skills they need to successfully cope with traumatic stress and adversity in early life.

This chapter reviews pediatric Posttraumatic Stress Disorder (PTSD), with a focus on children who experience multiple stressors and adversities. We discuss past research as well as our own published research and studies that are currently underway. Much of the research that we present is multimodal in approach and investigates areas including behavioral, emotional, anatomical, and biological aspects. We discuss how former research has influenced the novel treatments we have developed, such as our Cue-Centered Therapy approach, and large-scale preventive interventions such as the Health and Wellness Program, a yoga and mindfulness curriculum at schools. Integrated system models of primary and mental health are also introduced, including two examples that exist at the Ravenswood Family Health Center and The Center for Youth Wellness. This chapter aims to introduce pediatric PTSD to the general audience and inform that audience about current

O. Altamirano · V. G. Carrión (✉)
Department of Psychiatry and Behavioral Sciences, Early Life Stress and Pediatric Anxiety Program Stanford University, Stanford, CA, USA
e-mail: vcarrion@stanford.edu

© Springer International Publishing AG, part of Springer Nature 2018

J. G. Noll, I. Shalev (eds.), *The Biology of Early Life Stress*, Child Maltreatment Solutions Network, https://doi.org/10.1007/978-3-319-72589-5_6

practices aimed at helping to equip children with the skills they need to successfully adapt and overcome posttraumatic deficits.

6.1 Introduction to Trauma

There is a plethora of examples of traumatic events that people may be exposed to during a lifetime. Traumatic events can be man-made but can also include natural catastrophes outside of our control. Traumatic events can be very difficult to cope with, and children are even more vulnerable than adults to the effects of trauma. Hostile environments, such as a home marked with domestic abuse, are factors that children cannot control. As minors, they cannot simply change their living conditions. Moreover, children often have few and very basic coping skills, which may only be minimally effective when facing severe events. Additionally, children are often unable to cognitively appraise events as serious traumas and are thus less likely to seek resources when distressful events occur.

Man-made traumas include events such as the terrorist attacks of 9/11 and mass shootings in schools. Recent school shootings, where students are thought to be safe, include those at Virginia Polytechnic Institute and State University in Virginia in 2007 (Hauser & O'Connor, 2007), Sandy Hook Elementary School in Connecticut in 2012 (Vogel, Horwitz, & Fahrenthold, 2012), and Umpqua Community College in Oregon in 2015 (Vanderhart, Johnson, & Turkewitz, 2015), to name a few. On a smaller but no less significant scale, other man-made traumatic events include experiencing or witnessing physical abuse, sexual abuse, crimes, and accidents. Even in supportive family systems, some children may still be susceptible to these traumas in their larger communities.

Traumatic events can also come unexpectedly from natural forces. The 1989 Loma Prieta Earthquake in California left dozens dead and thousands wounded (History.com Staff, 2009). Over 1000 people died as a result of Hurricane Katrina in Louisiana (Rushton, 2015). People in Haiti have now experienced two of these natural disasters within 6 years: a 7.0 magnitude earthquake in 2010 and Hurricane Matthew in 2016 (Ansari, 2016). It is important to consider the possibility that in addition to the aforementioned natural traumas, some of these children could have also been exposed to other types of trauma, such as poverty or abuse. When combined, these factors paint an illustration of the potential accumulation of trauma.

6.1.1 Early Life Stress

McEwen and Tucker refer to the accumulation of stressors as the "allostatic load," which "confers some vulnerability to toxic exposures" (2011). They explain that allostatic load encompasses stressors such as low income, lack of education, vulnerable occupations, and chemical stressors (e.g., pollution and pesticides). The consideration of co-exposure in early life specifically renders allostatic loads potentially composed of: aggressive, irresponsible, or neglectful parenting; negative peer relationships; academic demands; and chronic family stress such as financial instability, concern for future prosperity, and adverse neighborhood conditions. The burden of all these stressors places children at risk to develop both physiological and psychological difficulties.

The following case offers a depiction of the allostatic load of 11-year-old Andy. Andy was referred to our clinic, the Early Life Stress and Pediatric Anxiety Program (ELSPAP), because he was becoming very aggressive with his siblings. His mom regarded this as something uncharacteristic of his usual demeanor. Furthermore, she reported he had decreased academic performance, frequent nightmares, and difficulty sleeping. After some time, Andy's mom disclosed that her partner had regularly abused the entire family, both physically and emotionally, for many years. Andy had been hit numerous times with metal bars, wooden rods, and bamboo sticks. Andy's mom blamed herself and thought that her son's behavior was directed at her for prompting the father's arrest and deportation, thus, "breaking the family up."

Andy was experiencing physical and emotional trauma, which led to poor academic achievement, a now conflict-laden relationship with his siblings and mom, and feelings of guilt. This is an example of the spiral that ensues when there is a history of trauma in a child's life. Trauma is not an isolated event; rather, there is usually secondary associated trauma, and these events have a concrete effect in the child's behavior and academic outcomes. We will continue to refer to Andy's story as the chapter continues.

Early life stress can impact many domains of life. For Andy, the impact was evident in his relationships, his sleep habits, and his academics. Research indicates that trauma is also correlated with suicidal ideation, anxiety, depression, and psychosis (Bendall, Alvarez- Jimenez, Hulbert, McGorry, & Jackson, 2012; Lansford et al., 2002; Thompson et al., 2012). The work at ELSPAP anchors on children's experiences of traumatic stress and how these lead to PTSD symptoms.

As classified by the American Psychological Association's *Diagnostic and Statistical Manual of Mental Disorders-5*, some of the criteria for PTSD in people older than 6 years of age include "exposure to actual or threatened death, serious injury, or sexual violence" (2013). Intrusion symptoms (e.g., distressing memories, flashbacks) and avoidance of stimuli are also noted in association to the traumatic event. One other criterion is negative changes in cognitions of the traumatic event (e.g., inability to recall parts of the traumatic event).

There is a belief that children are resilient by virtue of being children; the notion follows that somehow children are unaffected by stress. Research has not provided data to support this view. In fact, studies show the younger you are, the more vulnerable you can be (Thompson, 2014). Nonetheless, there are some children who may be exposed to trauma and will not be diagnosed with PTSD. Our field refers to undiagnosed children as "resilient," even though we have not yet fully conceptualized the term. People are currently categorized as resilient if they have not reached the threshold at which they show clinically diagnostic symptoms of functional impairment. In other words, being classified as resilient does not mean that they are unaffected; rather, they simply have not met diagnostic criteria.

Studies have published rates of PTSD among children who have experienced traumatic events to be between 10 and 50%; these rates might be higher if we take into account symptoms of PTSD (Cuffe et al., 1998). It is important to note that the above percentages do not include children who may have undiagnosed PTSD. There may be some families that are unable to observe the need for clinical care or cannot afford it and thus never receive a diagnosis or help. Further, the above percentages do not include children with large allostatic loads and elevated symptoms of PTSD that have not yet reached diagnostic levels. It is imperative, nonetheless, to also emphasize that children who do have subthreshold symptoms of PTSD often have similar impairments and levels of distress in comparison to those who meet full diagnostic criteria (Carrión, Weems, Ray, & Reiss, 2002).

As the trauma becomes more personal, such as physical, emotional, or sexual abuse, the prevalence rate for PTSD can be higher; one example of this is a 57.5% occurrence rate in one of our samples of children ages 5–17 (Kletter, Weems, & Carrión, 2009). From this, we can infer that there is a genetic proclivity for some individuals to be more vulnerable to the stress that very often accompanies traumatic experience. Essentially, we could all develop PTSD for certain events, such as kidnapping or torture; hence genetic proclivity could be overpowered by environmental experience. Some postulate that PTSD should not be considered a disorder at all and instead suggest the term Posttraumatic Stress Injury. Most injuries will progressively become worse if left untreated; for instance, a cut that is ignored may become infected and more difficult to heal. PTSD feeds on avoidance; therefore, the "approach" to it should be the answer.

6.1.2 Pediatric PTSD

The conceptualization of pediatric PTSD has been controversial. Currently, the DSM-5 has separate criteria for diagnosis among people age 6 and older and children younger than six. The cardinal feature of PTSD held in both distinctions is "… the development of characteristic symptoms following exposure to one or more traumatic events" (American Psychological Association, 2013, p. 274).

The data that we have gathered thus far shows that children do not necessarily have to qualify for diagnostic criteria in order to experience functional impairment. In other words, children can display functional impairment and remain undiagnosed because they have not met all the criteria or because they have simply not received mental health services. In order to quantify functional impairment, the field evaluates three domains: performance in school, relationships, and a child's own sense of distress. If none of the aforementioned domains are affected, then we consider the child not to have the disorder.

Some of the limitations of PTSD rely on its behaviorally defined approach. A movement has taken force in the past two decades to identify biological correlates of PTSD. These biological markers will help us better identify PTSD in children, provide more timely treatment, and help us create better interventions.

6.2 Goals for Pediatric PTSD Research

The Stanford Early Life Stress and Pediatric Anxiety Program's main overarching goal is to understand and address the effects of trauma on children. The following section will elucidate our team's goals in understanding pediatric trauma through scientific research, creating informed and innovative treatment models, developing predictors of treatment outcome, and helping advance clinical practice in this field.

6.2.1 Understanding the Pathogenesis of PTSD

Psychiatry and psychology have become more holistic in their perspective on early childhood development. There seems to be a consensus that the nature versus nurture debate is too dichotomous and that, in fact, both come together and shape the development of a child. These two are so intertwined that it would be logical to assume that diagnosis would inspect both innate and acquired symptoms. However, this is not true of our criteria for PTSD diagnosis, which currently lacks biological markers. Utilizing biological measures, in conjunction with already established behavioral ones, can guide more accurate and prompt diagnosis and consequently faster access to care.

6.2.2 Informing Treatments

One primary goal in conducting and learning from this research is to develop treatments and entice others to investigate and further the field as well. It is our informed opinion that treatment will likely be very specific to the experiences and behaviors of the children and that different circumstances will require a different approach. In other words, different types of trauma (e.g., interpersonal, natural event trauma) and subcategories of symptoms (e.g., self-injurious, non-self-injurious, dissociation) may be more responsive to one form of treatment than another. Therefore, it is vital for the field to develop more treatments for specific subgroups of youth with PTSD symptoms, a condition that is highly heterogeneous in its clinical presentation.

6.2.3 Discovering Predictors of Treatment Outcome

In addition to psychosocial and behavioral questionnaire assessments, we also focus on the biology of early life stress. By using a multimethod approach, we can investigate correlates between different domains that would have otherwise gone unnoticed if we had employed only one medium for assessment. In other words, we can learn about the associations among functional, anatomical, and biological measures, rather than the limited correlations garnered through only functional data. The following sections will provide information on some of the domains we are investigating in an attempt to better identify treatment outcomes.

6.2.3.1 Examining Cortisol

Sapolsky, Krey, and McEwen's (1986) work demonstrated that corticosterone, the stress hormone in rodents, can be neurotoxic to neural cells when at high levels. The investigators studied lab rats under stressors of, for example, exposure to cold. They found that younger rats were able to return their corticosterone levels to basal range within an hour after a stressor. Older rats that were under more chronic stress, on the other hand, showed an impaired ability to terminate the biological stress response, sometimes taking up to 24 h to return to normal levels. Moreover, the authors stated that cumulative exposure to stressors led to a deterioration of neurons and receptors located in the hippocampus of the rats. Further, they noted that chronic stressors, but not age necessarily, accelerate the neurodegenerative process. In sum, they observed that multiple stressors and stressors present for long periods of time reduced the number of neurons in the hippocampi of the laboratory rodents.

In response to those findings, we have examined cortisol developmentally in humans. Cortisol, known as a stress hormone in humans, is a window to the physiology of stress. Stress can be healthy; it can motivate us to meet deadlines and reach goals. However, while moderate levels of stress can be easily managed and channeled productively, the human body has its limits. Consider a young child who is constantly producing cortisol because he or she is constantly exposed to stressors. Although cortisol was necessary at one point, it may remain elevated even after the stressor is removed. If the neurodegenerative processes observed in rodents are similar for humans under multiple and chronic stress, this could have a severe impact on the developing child. Therefore, the consequences of dysregulated cortisol in human children must be investigated.

Our data published in 2009 shows a couple of differences between salivary cortisol in groups of children who reported interpersonal trauma and experienced PTSD symptoms and children without reported exposure to trauma (Weems & Carrión, 2009). When comparing the cortisol levels of children with PTSD symptoms to those without, we found that the decline from pre-breakfast collection to pre-lunch collection was steeper. Also, while the cortisol levels of the control group (those without reported trauma) decreased between pre-dinner and pre-bedtime, the levels of the children in the PTSD symptom group decreased significantly less. In other words, while the healthy control group experienced a decline in cortisol levels towards bedtime, the groups with PTSD symptoms showed a significantly higher pre-bedtime cortisol level.

It is interesting to consider some possibilities regarding children's difficulties at night time: they experience nightmares, fear of the dark, and enuresis (involuntary urination). Sleeping should be a time when people are relieved of their everyday responsibilities, a time to relax and recuperate, a time to become completely safe within one's environment. According to our data, however, children with pediatric posttraumatic stress symptoms demonstrate both behavioral nighttime difficulties and altered hormonal physiology.

We conceptualized PTSD as a developmental disorder and were inclined to study this biologically. First, by defining PTSD as a "developmental disorder" we are suggesting that this is a disorder in which time since the trauma, and time since the symptoms started, is taken into account. How long does a stressor have to insult the body until it affects it? PTSD is not something that remains static; it changes. It can be ameliorated through treatment or worsened through avoidance. Consider a 10-year-old child who has been living with undiagnosed PTSD since age 5, and a 35-year-old who has recently experienced trauma. Although younger, the child will present a more chronic physiological picture.

In 2007, we conducted a study aimed at identifying the role that time plays in PTSD (Weems & Carrión). We assessed the cortisol levels for children in one of two groups: one consisting of children who had experienced trauma within the last year, and a second consisting of children whose trauma experience had occurred over one year ago. As in our previous studies, cortisol was elevated for those children who had PTSD symptoms, but only for those who had experienced the recent events. Conversely, when the event was more distal, we observed lower levels of pre-bedtime cortisol. This may reflect autoregulation of the axis responsible for cortisol secretion, or decreased sensitivity for the regulating system. There is a concern that high levels of cortisol may be neurotoxic to sensitive areas of the brain that have glucocorticoid receptors (receptors that bind to cortisol), such as the hippocampus and the prefrontal cortex (PFC). Both structures are involved in functions that become dysregulated in PTSD: namely, memory and executive function. The hippocampus, for example, a structure within the medial temporal lobe, is involved in our memory encoding and retrieval (Squire & Zola-Morgan, 1991).

6.2.3.2 Examining Brain Structure and Function Via Magnetic Resonance Imaging (MRI)

High-resolution imaging allows us to accurately determine volumetric measurements of the brain and does not require radiation or contrast, making this a safe method to use with children. Data published by Shimamura (2000) has shown that irregularities of the PFC can prompt obstacles to attention, memory, and emotion regulation.

In 2007 we examined, in a longitudinal pilot study, the correlations between pre-bedtime cortisol levels and hippocampal volumes (Carrión, Weems, Reiss). Cross-sectional studies had not demonstrated any hippocampal changes. Believing the process of neurotoxicity to be pernicious, we followed children with PTSD symptoms for a year and a half to examine a potential association between pre-bedtime cortisol levels and hippocampal volumes. We observed that between baseline and the 12-month and 18-month follow-ups, a hippocampal decrease was predicted by a stronger severity of PTSD symptoms and higher pre-bedtime cortisol levels (Carrión, Weems, & Reiss, 2007). This was the first published study to show correlations between cortisol, a biological marker, and hippocampal changes in a group with posttraumatic stress symptoms.

We followed this study with a controlled fMRI study examining hippocampal function with a memory task. The healthy control group demonstrated significantly more hippocampal activity during the memory task (Carrión, Haas, Garret, Song, & Reiss, 2010). Participants were trained on a verbal declarative memory task and were instructed to identify words that had been presented previously from a group of old and new words. We observed increased activity of the hippocampus in the control group compared to the group with posttraumatic stress symptoms.

In 2010, we investigated brain tissue and cerebral gray matter, by means of MRI, in a sample of 30 youth who had experienced trauma and 15 youth who did not report trauma (Carrión, Weems, Richert, Hoffman, & Reiss). We observed the PTSD symptom group to have a significantly smaller amount of brain tissue and cerebral gray matter in the PFC than the group without reported trauma. This suggests that children with PTSD symptoms experience concrete differences in brain anatomy: they have less brain tissue and less gray matter. We also analyzed cortisol levels collected from both of the aforementioned groups. A significantly negative correlation was found between pre-bedtime cortisol levels and the left ventral PFC volumes. Specifically, those children that had the highest levels of cortisol at night also had a lower volume of gray matter on the ventral PFC.

We followed the PFC findings with an fMRI study utilizing an executive function task, the Go/No-Go (Carrión, Garret, Menon, Weems, & Reiss, 2008). Imagine a black screen with letters appearing in the middle, one at a time. The participant's task is to press a mouse with his pointer finger every time he sees a letter and not to press when the letter "X" appears. Initially, we had hypothesized for this study that the children with PTSD might be more impulsive than the group without PTSD symptoms, which was age and gender matched. The data showed instead that both groups performed similarly behaviorally; in other words, they were pressing at about the same rates. This observation allows us to safely conclude that the differences that we observed were neurofunctional differences not associated with their behavioral performance; instead, the resulting differences can be attributed to neurofunctional correlates of executive function.

The results show that the participants in the control group, healthy children with no history of trauma, and the group with PTSD symptoms are appropriately activating areas such as the superior, middle, and inferior parts of the frontal cortex (Carrión et al., 2008). The control group was, however, activating the medial frontal cortex significantly more than the PTSD group. A reverse analysis of the data showed the group with PTSD symptoms activated the medial PFC; interestingly, this area is not meant to be activated by this "Go/No-Go" task. The primary role of the medial PCF is to manage and process emotional information. Additional analysis showed that this activation was related to comorbidity and the presence of anxiety, an interesting area for future research.

In order to address heterogeneity in PTSD, we split the PTSD participants into two groups: those with a history of self-injurious behaviors and those with no such history (Carrión et al., 2008). The data from the Go/No-Go task showed that the group of participants who engaged in self-injurious behaviors had significantly increased activity in the insula compared to the group who did not engage in these behaviors. In fact, there was a very strong and direct correlation between the total task score, PTSD symptoms, and activation of the insula. The insula is a cortical region in the temporal lobe that is involved in processing somatic (i.e., sensory) information; it receives input and helps deliver information to different parts of the body. These results suggest a neurofunctional marker for deficits in executive function in the PTSD group in the middle frontal lobe and increased involvement of the temporal lobe with increased PTSD symptoms.

Thus far, we have reviewed two tasks examining cognitive function: executive function and memory. We later conducted an emotion task during which 46 participants viewed emotionally expressive faces and were asked to press buttons that were indicative of the sex portrayed by the face (Garret et al., 2012). We observed an early activation of the amygdala when the PTSD symptom participants were presented with angry faces, while the same activation was not observed in the control group. This was an interesting finding in that it was contrary to the initial hypothesis. We had originally postulated that we were going to see activation of the amygdala when we presented fearful faces, not angry ones. In examining the relationship, we noted that our PTSD symptom participants had a history of interpersonal violence and physical abuse at home. Thus, their cue was not seeing fearful faces; their cue was actually being approached by someone who appeared angry. According to this study, heightened amygdala activity could be a neurofunctional marker for hyperarousability. By considering the environments these children often live in, we can attempt to explain this hyperarousability. These children live in places where it is important for them to be able to properly and quickly rate the safety or danger of their environment. Given this context, hyperarousability can be adaptive. The issue arises when children are not able to come down from this hyperaroused state into a more relaxed one; they are constantly and relentlessly expecting danger. These children lack the cognitive flexibility to know when this skill is necessary and when it is not. For example, if one of these participants is in a classroom that becomes very loud, this can be a reminder of the level of noise experienced at home if there is domestic violence. If this is the case, the child might be tempted to run out of the classroom if escaping this type of situation at home has proven helpful before. Unfortunately, it is likely that this student will be incorrectly labeled as a "behavior problem" and that his or her situation will not be considered in context of the child's experience.

6.3 Cue-Centered Therapy (CCT)

The above observations that trauma can have a negative effect on cognitive, emotional, physiological, and behavioral domains led us to develop a short-term (15-session) individual form of treatment modality named Cue-Centered Therapy (CCT) (Carrión, 2016). CCT is a hybrid form of treatment that successfully combines elements of cognitive, behavioral, psychodynamic, expressive, and family therapies (Carrión, Kletter, Weems, Berry, & Rettger, 2013). This particular treatment was designed primarily for youth who have experienced traumatic events, including the aforementioned man-made and natural disasters, physical and sexual abuse, and exposure to violence, and who are concurrently and chronically facing environmental adversity.

CCT builds the child's empowerment through knowledge and active participation in the treatment. For example, after some training, he or she will choose the cues that will anchor the therapy. Recognizing that families that experience chronic adversity have difficulties engaging in ongoing treatment, CCT limits the caregiver involvement requirement to four sessions in which caregiver and child are both able to recognize, understand, and learn how to practice the objectives of the therapy at home.

Anxiety and depression have been found to be of comorbidity as high as 80% in people with PTSD (Pfefferbaum, 1997). A randomized controlled trial (RCT) provided data suggesting that CCT can lower symptoms of both disorders (Carrión et al., 2013). Moreover, the RCT showed a decrease in PTSD symptoms when measured both by self-report and by caregivers (Carrión et al., 2013). In order to better illustrate this model, we will consider Andy, the child we introduced in Sect. 6.1.1.

6.3.1 CCT and Cognition

With CCT, the child gains insight into his or her history and into how previous exposures to traumatic events may be affecting present experiences, thus resulting in maladaptive behaviors (Carrión et al., 2013). Children receiving this treatment are introduced to the idea of allostatic load, which we discussed earlier in the chapter (Sect. 6.1.1). With the help of a therapist, the children identify traumatic events and use a timeline as a visual representation of these and other daily stressors. In building this timeline, a child is able to visualize a personal narration of events that had a large impact on his or her life.

Through CCT, Andy learned the meaning of trauma, principles of classical conditioning, and PTSD symptoms and was able to identify his own cues. Andy also learned that it was normal for someone with trauma to have discordant feelings and that it was completely understandable that he missed his father while simultaneously feeling safer now that his dad was not hitting him or the family. Even though he was initially resistant, Andy was able to implement the relaxation strategies that he learned, which gave him a sense of control and a feeling of calmness.

Instead of trying to change Andy's appraisal of the trauma, we attempted to balance his negative intrusive thoughts with information and perspectives gathered about his strengths. On the other hand, we can try to change rigid cognitive distortions. We use reframing and reattribution of these distortions by drawing from the child's own narratives about other events in which he or she acted in a way that is not endorsed by the cognitive distortion.

Through CCT, we also teach the children emotion regulation skills. Cognitive processing therapy has been adapted and used with children who experience trauma (Silverman et al., 2008) and is designed to help them modify their appraisal of the trauma, given the context of their ongoing lives (Cohen, Perel, De Bellis, Friedman, & Putnam, 2002). We emphasized the need for children to be able to identify and express their feelings. Many times, children will use very broad words to describe their feelings, for example "I felt bad." Instead of trying to elaborate for the child, the CCT therapists' role is to help the child elaborate on his or her own by asking open-ended questions in order to avoid influencing responses.

6.3.2 CCT and Behavior

Part of CCT is modeled after behavioral exposure techniques. These have been proven helpful in a variety of studies involving PTSD by lessening depressive symptoms, disrupting the trigger association, and decreasing avoidance (Cohen, Mannarino, Berliner, & Deblinger, 2000; Silva et al., 2003; Smith et al., 2013). In CCT, we use a few different approaches to gradually expose the child to the cues: imaginary exposure, in-session exposure, and an in-vivo exposure assignment.

After a few sessions, when the child has gained insight and has been able to identify cues, we introduce imaginary exposure. By imagining the cue, the child is able to abstain from the negative consequences that are typically catastrophized. Instead, this imaginary exposure allows the child to mindfully witness his or her responses to it, such as increased heart rate and sweating. This further allows the child to recognize a disproportionate response to a given cue. For Andy, one cue was the slamming of the car door. This sound was associated with aggression and reminded him of many fights between his parents and of instances in which his drunken father would physically assault him and his family. In imaginary exposure, the therapist might instruct Andy to think about all the details of the car and to then think of its door being slammed by his parent. The therapist would then proceed to help Andy identify his body's reaction to the imaginary sound.

Next, the child has an opportunity to experience cues while role playing situations with the therapist that may otherwise provoke stressful responses when experienced outside of the therapeutic session. Essentially, in-session exposure allows the child to experience the cues and act out a scenario in a more direct way than imaginary exposure, while also easing the way towards the more vivid trigger. This role play allows for the child to engage in some of the coping skills that he or she has learned in CCT in a safe environment and provides a way to familiarize and make the child feel comfortable with employing these skills. For Andy, this exposure might entail slamming the door at the therapists' office. He and the therapist would then brainstorm coping techniques, such as relaxed breathing, in order to alleviate his reaction.

Last, the child is able to use the skills learned thus far and incorporate the imaginary and in-session cues to manage an increasingly more challenging in-vivo exposure. This exposure is assigned to the children to be conducted at home. In-vivo exposure allows the child to gain self-efficacy in order to successfully employ the skills in future stressful situations, which are likely to continue after therapy services have concluded. Once the assignment is complete, the therapist conducts a session around that assignment. A dialogue is maintained with the child to learn from the original response and generate even more adaptive responses to employ in the future. Andy and his therapist might talk in this session about witnessing his mother slam the door and how Andy reacted to it. For instance, it is possible that he practiced relaxed breathing. The therapist would applaud Andy's coping strategy and further suggest that he also come up with a larger repertoire of responses in the case that this single technique does not alleviate his feelings.

6.4 Treatment Outcome Research

Individual therapy is very helpful, and we are determined to make the skills practiced in individual therapy more accessible to large groups of children. We sought to teach children these skills early so that if they experienced trauma, they would already have the skills to avert trauma's detrimental effects. In order to avoid stigma and develop an accessible and affordable plan (Jaycox, Stein, & Amaya-Jackson, 2009), we decided that a school-based approach would be best suited for our targeted population. Specifically, we aimed to disseminate programs that helped children to cope with adversity by focusing on emotion regulation and executive function.

6.4.1 The Health and Wellness Study

The purpose of the Health and Wellness Study Program is to intervene early and increase coping methods. Earlier, in Sect. 6.2.3.2: *Examining Brain Structure and Function via MRI*, we discussed regions of the brain that seem to be affected by environmental stressors and trauma, including the prefrontal cortex. While these areas are difficult to investigate and interpret, they seem to be some of the most plastic regions. Therefore, we designed a curriculum that teaches children emotion regulation skills and strengthens their executive functioning. In an effort to protect children from later stressors, we attempt to provide a supportive and understanding environment that may reverse or hinder the effect of chronic stress. In order to increase the accessibility and affordability of interventions to a diverse population, we decided to implement this at a school level (Berger, Pat-Horenczyk, & Gelkopf, 2007).

We approached the Ravenswood City School District (RCSD) in East Palo Alto, CA, an area that has historically been under-resourced and high in crime; it was at one point the number-one murder capital in the United States (Warren, 1993). In partnership with Pure Edge Incorporated, we developed a mindfulness and yoga curriculum that RCSD students are now receiving two to three times a week, beginning in kindergarten and lasting through eighth grade. Mindfulness can help children strengthen their executive functioning skills by encouraging them to monitor and sustain their concentration (Flook et al., 2010). Yoga adds on a physical component and has also been shown to produce benefits for executive function tasks (Manjunath & Telles, 2001). The curriculum comprises breathing exercises, posture exercises, nutrition education, and coping skills.

6.4.1.1 Evaluating the Effectiveness of the Health and Wellness Study

Earlier, we stated the importance of a multimethod approach (Sect. 6.2.3); this is our approach to the evaluation of the Health and Wellness Program. Our participants allow us to collect a variety of assessments in this biopsychosocial study, including: salivary cortisol samples; neuroimaging scans; polysomnography tests; behavioral, emotional, intellectual functioning tests; and academic data. We are able to learn about the children's cortisol levels, brain anatomy and functioning, sleep quality, behavioral characteristics, emotions, learning abilities, grades, and truancies, among other things. In the analysis, we will be able to look at the relationships among all of these domains.

Further, we are working with a nearby school district to act as a control (not receiving the intervention), as it serves very similar students demographically, socio-economically, and in terms of adversity. This partnership will allow us to make between-group comparisons in the evaluation of this intervention when compared to a control group. The goal of this information is to gather three-year longitudinal data in order to make strong developmental correlations.

6.5 Policy

While conducting and publishing studies has been productive, we feel that a necessary second step of translation is disseminating evidence-based interventions. Our research should impact clinical practice but should also inform policy. Bronfenbrenner's ecological system model provides an outline for the influences during children's development (1977). He defines the microsystem as being composed of activities associated with the innermost circle of the child's life, including the parents, school, and friends. He then goes on to explain the next outer layer, the mesosystem, which he describes as being composed of the relationships between the entities in the child's microsystem, e.g., the relationship between the parent and the child's teacher. We want to impact more than just those two systems; we also want to impact the exosystem. Bronfenbrenner describes the exosystem as consisting of the social institutions that have indirect effects on children (1977). In order to have an impact at that level, we are participating in two programs that are aimed at integrating primary and mental health: The Center for Youth Wellness and Ravenswood Family Health Center.

6.5.1 Center for Youth Wellness

In 2007, we began a multidisciplinary partnership with other individuals and institutions with the aim to provide innovative, trauma-informed care to people in the community experiencing chronic stress and trauma. Five years later, in 2012, we founded the Center for Youth Wellness in the community of Bayview Hunter's Point in southeast San Francisco, CA (Walker & Carrión, 2015). This community has experienced high rates of trauma and adversity, including economic difficulties, community violence, institutionalized racism, and environmental toxins, to name a few (Katz, 2006). In order to address these needs, we at Stanford Early Life Stress and Pediatric Anxiety Program partnered with multiple organizations including the Tipping Point Community, the University of California, San Francisco's Child Trauma Research Program, the San Francisco Child Abuse Prevention Center's Children's Advocacy Center, and Bayview Health Center. We also sought to include people living in the community by forming a community advisory council that was open not only to direct participants but also to neighborhood residents (Walker & Carrión, 2015).

At the Center for Youth Wellness, patients will find two organizations in one building: Bayview Child Health Center and the Children's Advocacy Center. When families come in for primary care—for example, a pediatric checkup at the Bayview Child Health Center—the CYW screens the children for Adverse Childhood Experiences (ACEs). Briefly, the ACE study was conducted by the Kaiser Foundation and assessed the presence of categories including physical and emotional abuse and neglect, sexual abuse, and traumas involving the person's direct inner circle (Felitti et al., 1998). The researchers found that as the amount of endorsed ACEs increased, so did the risk for chronic disease in adulthood. Patients can also receive mental health services and therapy, including CCT.

6.5.2 Ravenswood Family Health Center

In 2008, Ravenswood Family Health Center (RFHC) created Integrated Behavioral Health Services (IBHS), novel in part for placing fellows and clinicians of child and adolescent psychiatry in the community (Aguirre & Carrión, 2012). Data gathered the year prior to the aforementioned publication showed that RFHC patients consisted of 40% aged less than 18, 73% Latino, and 90% living under the federal poverty line (Aguirre & Carrión, 2012).

IBHS aims to help youth who are experiencing or are at risk for behavioral challenges by providing brief psychosocial services, typically between one and five sessions, in an effort to help as many patients as possible (Aguirre & Carrión, 2012). Moreover, this model strives to implement early intervention, to engage pediatricians and behavioral health workers, and to provide effective and brief treatment. Referrals from pediatricians are made to IBHS when the identifying issues are present as developmental barriers that can be briefly treated. In other words, if the case merits longer-term and more involved therapy, referrals will be made outside of the clinic. Examples of the kinds of issues treated at this facility range from children presenting behavioral issues at school to youth who have experienced domestic violence. The data we collected showed that pediatricians are highly satisfied with the availability and quality of the services provided by IBHS and that they consider the services provided as critical.

6.6 Summary

PTSD can be harmful to a developing child because it affects many domains of life including interpersonal relationships and academics. Research also shows that the effects of trauma on children can have concrete anatomical and biological consequences (Carrión et al., 2007; Weems & Carrión, 2009). For these reasons, it is imperative to intervene early and to teach children the skills they will need if they are faced with trauma.

We want to work collaboratively to empower children and equip them to be their own agents of change. It is vital that they feel empowered to exert control over their responses to stress, and we hope to be creating a pathway in that direction. By disseminating treatments informed by research, we hope to give young children the resources they need for successful lives.

References

Aguirre, J., & Carrión, V. G. (2012). Integrated behavioral health services: A collaborative care model for pediatric patients in a low-income setting. *Clinical Pediatrics, 52*(12), 1178–1180. https://doi.org/10.1177/0009922812470744

American Psychiatric Association. (2013). *Diagnostic and statistical manual of mental disorders* (5th ed.). Washington, DC, Author.

Ansari, A. (2016, October 8). *Hurricane Matthew: Death Toll Rising in Haiti*. CNN. Retrieved from http://www.cnn.com/2016/10/08/americas/hurricane-matthew-death-toll-haiti/

Bendall, S., Alvarez- Jimenez, M., Hulbert, C. A., McGorry, P. D., & Jackson, H. J. (2012). Childhood trauma increases the risk of post- traumatic stress disorder in response to first- episode psychosis. *The Australian and New Zealand Journal of Psychiatry, 46*(1), 35–39. https://doi.org/10.1177/0004867411430877

Berger, R., Pat-Horenczyk, R., & Gelkopf, M. (2007). School-based intervention for prevention and treatment of elementary-students' terror-related distress in Israel: A quasi-randomized controlled trial. *Journal of Traumatic Stress, 20*, 541–551. https://doi.org/10.1002/jts.20225

Brofenbrenner, U. (1977). Toward an experimental ecology of human development. *American Psychologist, 32*(7), 513–531.

Carrión, V. G. (2016). *Cue-centered therapy for youth experiencing posttraumatic symptoms: A structured, multimodal intervention, therapist guide*. New York, NY: Oxford University Press.

Carrión, V. G., Garret, A., Menon, V., Weems, C. F., & Reiss, A. L. (2008). Posttraumatic stress symptoms and brain functioning during a response- inhibition task: An fMRI study in youth. *Depression and Anxiety, 25*, 514–526.

Carrión, V. G., Haas, B. W., Garret, A. G., Song, S., & Reiss, A. L. (2010). Reduced hippocampal activity in youth with posttraumatic stress symptoms: An fMRI study. *Journal of Pediatric Psychology, 35*(5), 559–569.

Carrión, V. G., Kletter, H., Weems, C. F., Berry, R. R., & Rettger, J. P. (2013). Cue-centered treatment for youth exposed to interpersonal violence: A randomized controlled trial. *Journal of Traumatic Stress, 26*, 654–662. https://doi.org/10.1002/jts.21870

Carrión, V. G., Weems, C. F., Ray, R., & Reiss, A. L. (2002). Toward an empirical definition of pediatric PTSD: The phenomenology of PTSD symptoms in youth. *Journal of the American Academy of Child and Adolescent Psychiatry, 41*(2), 166–173.

Carrión, V. G., Weems, C. F., & Reiss, A. L. (2007). Stress predicts brain changes in children: A pilot longitudinal study on youth stress, posttraumatic stress disorder, and the hippocampus. *Pediatrics, 19*(3), 509–516. https://doi.org/10.1542/peds.2006-2028

Carrión, V. G., Weems, C. F., Richert, K. A., Hoffman, B. C., & Reiss, A. L. (2010). Decreased prefrontal cortical volume associated with increased bedtime cortisol in traumatized youth. *Biological Psychiatry, 68*(5), 491–493. https://doi.org/10.1016/j.biopsych.2010.05.010

Cohen, J., Perel, J. M., De Bellis, M. D., Friedman, M. J., & Putnam, F. W. (2002). Treating traumatized children: Clinical implications of the psychobiology of posttraumatic stress disorder. *Trauma, Violence, and Abuse: A Review Journal, 3*(2), 91–108. https://doi.org/10.1177/15248380020032001

Cohen, J. A., Mannarino, A. P., Berliner, L., & Deblinger, E. (2000). Trauma-focused cognitive behavioral therapy for children and adolescents: An empirical update. *Journal of Interpersonal Violence, 15*(11), 1202–1223.

Cuffe, S. P., Addy, C. L., Garrison, C. Z., Waller, J. L., Jackson, K. L., McKeown, R. E., & Chilappagari, S. (1998). Prevelance of PTSD in a community sample of older adolescents. *Journal of the American Academy of Child and Adolescent Psychiatry, 37*(2), 147–154.

Felitti, V. J., Anda, R. F., Nordenberg, D., Williamson, D. F., Spitz, A. M., Edwards, V., … Marks, J. S. (1998). Relationship of childhood abuse and household dysfunction to many of the leading causes of death in adults: The Adverse Childhood Experiences (ACE) study. *American Journal of Preventive Medicine, 14*(4), 245–258.

Flook, L., Smalley, S. L., Kitil, M. J., Galla, B. M., Kaiser-Greenland, S., Locke, J., … Kasari, C. (2010). Effects of mindful awareness practices on executive functions in elementary school children. *Journal of Applied School Psychology, 26*(1), 70–95. https://doi.org/10.1080/15377900903379125

Garret, A. S., Carrión, V. G., Kletter, H., Karchemskiy, A., Weems, C. F., & Reiss, A. (2012). Brain activation to facial expressions in youth with PTSD symptoms. *Depression and Anxiety, 29*, 449–459. https://doi.org/10.1002/da.21892

Hauser, C., & O'Connor, A. (2007, April 16). Virginia Tech shooting leaves 33 dead. *The New York Times*. Retrieved from http://www.nytimes.com/2007/04/16/us/16cnd-shooting.html?_r=0

History.com Staff. (2009). 1989 San Francisco earthquake. History. Retrieved from http://www.history.com/topics/1989-san-francisco-earthquake

Jaycox, L. H., Stein, B. D., & Amaya-Jackson, L. (2009). School-based treatment for children and adolescents. In E. B. Foa, T. M. Keane, M. J. Friedman, & J. A. Cohen (Eds.), *Effective treatments for PTSD: Practice guidelines from the international society for traumatic stress studies* (2nd ed., pp. 327–345). New York, NY: Guilford Press.

Katz, M. H. (2006). *Health programs in Bayview Hunter's Point and recommendations for improving the health of Bayview Hunter's point residents*. San Francisco, CA: San Francisco Department of Public Health, Office of Policy and Planning.

Kletter, H., Weems, C. F., & Carrión, V. G. (2009). Guilt and posttraumatic stress symptoms in child victims of interpersonal violence. *Clinical Child Psychology and Psychiatry, 14*(1), 71–83. https://doi.org/10.1177/1359104508100137

Lansford, J. E., Dodge, K. A., Pettit, G. S., Bates, J. E., Crozier, J., & Kaplow, J. (2002). A 12-year prospective study of the long term effects of early child physical maltreatment on psychological, behavioral, and academic problems in adolescence. *Archives of Pediatrics and Adolescent Medicine, 156*(8), 824–830.

Manjunath, N. K., & Telles, S. (2001). Improved performance in the tower of London test following yoga. *Indian Journal of Physiology and Pharmacology, 45*(3), 351–354.

McEwen, B. S., & Tucker, P. (2011, September 1). Critical biological pathways for chronic psychosocial stress and research opportunities to advance the consideration of stress in chemical risk assessment. *American Journal of Public Health, 101*, S131–S139. https://doi.org/10.2105/AJPH.2011.300270

Pfefferbaum, B. (1997). Posttraumatic stress disorder in children: A review of the past 10 years. *Journal of the American Academy of Child & Adolescent Psychiatry, 36*, 1503–1511.

Rushton, C. (2015, August 28). Timeline: Hurricane Katrina and the aftermath. USA Today. Retrieved from http://www.usatoday.com/story/news/nation/2015/08/24/timeline-hurricane-katrina-and-aftermath/32003013/

Sapolsky, R. M., Krey, L. C., & McEwen, B. S. (1986). The neuroendocrinology of stress and aging: The glucorticoid cascade hypothesis. *Endocrine Reviews, 7*(3), 284–301. https://doi.org/10.1210/edrv-7-3-284

Shimamura, A. P. (2000). The role of the prefrontal cortex in dynamic filtering. *Psychobiology, 28*(2), 207–218.

Silva, R. R., Cloitra, M., Davis, L., Levitt, J., Gomez, S., Ngai, I., & Brown, E. (2003). Early intervention with traumatized children. *Psychiatric Quarterly, 74*(4), 333–347.

Silverman, W. K., Ortiz, C. D., Viswesvaran, C., Burns, B. J., Kolko, D. J., Putnam, F. W., & Amaya-Jackson, L. (2008). Evidence-based psychosocial treatments for children and adolescents exposed to traumatic events. *Journal of Clinical Child and Adolescent Psychology, 37*(1), 156–183.

Smith, P., Perrin, S., Dalgleish, T., Meiser-Stedman, R., Clark, D. M., & Yule, W. (2013). Treatment of posttraumatic stress disorder in children and adolescents. *Current Opinion in Psychiatry, 26*(1), 66–72.

Squire, L. R., & Zola-Morgan, S. (1991). The medial temporal lobe memory system. *Science, 254*, 1091–1099.

Thompson, R., Proctor, L. J., English, D. J., Dubowitz, H., Narasimhan, S., & Everson, M. D. (2012). Suicidal ideation in adolescence: Examining the role of recent adverse experiences. *Journal of Adolescence, 35*, 175–186. https://doi.org/10.1016/j.adolescence,2011.03.003

Thompson, R. A. (2014). Stress and child development. *The Future of Children, 24*(1), 41–59. https://doi.org/10.1353/foc.2014.0004

Vanderhart, D., Johnson, K., & Turkewitz, J. (2015, October 1). Oregon shooting at Umpqua College kills 10, sheriff says. *The New York Times*. Retrieved from http://www.nytimes.com/2015/10/02/us/oregon-shooting-umpqua-community-college.html

Vogel, S., Horwitz, S., & Fahrenthold, D. A. (2012, December 14). Sandy hook elementary shooting leaves 28 dead, law enforcement sources say. *The Washington Post*. Retrieved from https://www.washingtonpost.com/politics/sandy-hook-elementary-school-shooting-leaves-students-staff-dead/2012/12/14/24334570-461e-11e2-8e70-e1993528222d_story.html

Walker, S. E., & Carrión, V. G. (2015). Narrative 3: The center for youth wellness: A community-based approach to holistic health care in San Francisco. In L. W. Roberts, D. Reicherter, S. Adelsheim, & S. Joshi (Eds.), *Partnerships for mental health: Narratives of community and academic collaboration* (pp. 37–51). Cham: Springer International.

Warren, J. (1993, January 05). E. Palo Alto murder rate worst in U.S.; Drug wars blamed. *Los Angeles Times*. Retrieved from: http://articles.latimes.com/1993-01-05/local/me-833_1_east-palo-alto

Weems, C. F., & Carrión, V. G. (2009). Brief report: Diurnal salivary cortisol in youth—clarifying the nature of posttraumatic stress dysregulation. *Journal of Pediatric Psychology, 34*(4), 389–395. https://doi.org/10.1093/jpepsy/jsn087

Chapter 7
Epigenetics and Early Life Adversity: Current Evidence and Considerations for Epigenetic Studies in the Context of Child Maltreatment

Andrée-Anne Bouvette-Turcot, Michael J. Meaney, and Kieran J. O'Donnell

Profound developmental origins exist for individual differences in mental health that extend over the lifespan. Studies of institutionalization (McGoron et al., 2012; McLaughlin et al., 2013; Nelson et al., 2007; Rutter, Kumsta, Schlotz, & Sonuga-Barke, 2012) and childhood abuse (Nanni, Uher, & Danese, 2012; Trickett, Noll, & Putnam, 2011; Widom, DuMont, & Czaja, 2007) reflect the profound influence of the early social environment on development and mental health. Importantly, child maltreatment not only predicts the risk for multiple mental disorders, but at least in the case of depression, also the severity and treatment response (Nanni et al., 2012).

An obvious question concerns the mechanism by which the effects of the early environment become embedded in the molecular machinery that then regulates genomic function. In this chapter, we examine the evidence for the environmental epigenetics hypothesis, which proposes that the sustained effects of environmental conditions on gene expression are mediated by epigenetics mechanisms. We also discuss the current status of translational research that examines the role of epigenetics in the context of studies of child development. Additionally, we evaluate the clinical relevance of epigenetics for child/adolescent mental health and highlight considerations for future studies, which seek to incorporate epigenetic measures in studies with maltreated youth.

A.-A. Bouvette-Turcot (✉) · M. J. Meaney · K. J. O'Donnell
Douglas Mental Health University Institute, Montreal, QC, Canada

Department of Psychiatry, McGill University, Montreal, QC, Canada
e-mail: andree-anne.bouvette-turcot@mail.mcgill.ca; kieran.odonnell@mcgill.ca

© Springer International Publishing AG, part of Springer Nature 2018
J. G. Noll, I. Shalev (eds.), *The Biology of Early Life Stress*, Child Maltreatment Solutions Network, https://doi.org/10.1007/978-3-319-72589-5_7

7.1 Epigenetics

When we think of genomic influences, we most commonly imagine effects associated with variations in nucleotide sequence such as single nucleotide polymorphisms (SNPs). Yet such variations are only one form of information contained within the genome. Despite the reverence afforded DNA, a gene is basically like any other molecule in the cell; it is subject to modifications that change both its structure and function. Epigenetics, stemming from the Greek "*epi*" meaning "upon" and "*genetics*," refers to a series of chemical modifications to DNA and/or the proteins DNA is wrapped around, collectively referred to as *chromatin*.

For reasons of graphic simplicity, we often describe the organization of a gene or the interactions between DNA and proteins that regulate gene expression (transcription factors) as if the DNA were a linear molecule to which transcription factors gain unimpeded access. The reality of protein–DNA interactions is very different. DNA is commonly organized in a form that resembles beads lying along a string. The beads are nucleosomes, which consist of ~146 base pairs of DNA wrapped around a core of histone proteins (Turner, 2001). The histones and DNA together are referred to as chromatin; the nucleosome is one unit of chromatin.

Under normal conditions, a tight physical relation exists between the histone proteins and their accompanying DNA, resulting in a closed nucleosome configuration. This restrictive configuration is maintained, in part, by electrostatic bonds between the positively charged histones and the negatively charged DNA. The closed configuration impedes transcription factor binding and is associated with a reduced level of gene expression. Epigenetic modifications essentially favor either a closed or open state of chromatin. The functional significance of such modifications lies in the degree to which chromatin structure gates the ability of transcription factors to bind to DNA and activate transcription, which leads to gene expression. A closed nucleosome disfavors transcription factor binding and associates with transcriptional silencing. An increase in transcription factor binding to DNA, and the subsequent activation of gene expression, commonly requires chemical modification of the chromatin that occurs on the histone proteins. These modifications alter chromatin in a manner that either increases or decreases the ability of transcription factors to access regulatory sites on the DNA that control gene transcription.

The dynamic alteration of chromatin structure is achieved in part through covalent modifications to the histone proteins at the amino acids that form the histone protein tails that extend out from the nucleosome. There are several examples of such modifications, including but not limited to acetylation, phosphorylation, methylation, and ubiquitylation (see Maze, Noh, & Allis, 2013). In addition to these chemical modifications, histone proteins at the center of a nucleosome have multiple subtypes (e.g., H2A, H2B, and H3 variants), which influence the structure and function of surrounding DNA (Skene & Henikoff, 2013).

7.1.1 DNA Methylation

Another level of regulation occurs not on the histone proteins but directly on the DNA. Indeed, the classic epigenetic alteration is that of DNA methylation, which involves the addition of a methyl group (CH_3) onto cytosines predominately bound to guanines (CpGs) in the DNA (Bird, 1986; Holliday, 1989; Razin & Riggs, 1980; Razin & Cedar, 1993). DNA methylation can also occur on cytosines followed by a non-guanine base, which is referred to as non-CG or CpH methylation. Non-CG methylation is especially abundant in pluripotent stem cells and within the brain (Lister et al., 2013); however, the relevance of non-CG methylation for child neurodevelopment is yet to be established.

DNA methylation in the promoter region of a gene is typically associated with transcriptional repression, although the relationship between DNA methylation and transcription is context-dependent. For example, DNA methylation outside of the gene promoter, such as in the gene body, can be positively associated with gene expression (Maunakea et al., 2010; Shenker & Flanagan, 2012). The repressive effect of DNA methylation on gene transcription appears to be mediated in one of two ways (Bird, 2002). First, wide swaths of densely methylated DNA preclude transcription factor binding to DNA sites, thus silencing gene expression. The second manner is subtler and probably far more prevalent in regions with more dynamic variations in gene transcription, such as the brain. In this case, selected cytosines are methylated, and the presence of the methyl group attracts a class of proteins known as methylated-DNA binding proteins (Klose & Bird, 2006). These proteins, in turn, attract an entire cluster of proteins that form a repressor complex, which includes active mediators of gene silencing.

DNA demethylation associates with a return to an open, euchromatin state, which occurs subsequent to specific histone modifications (Weaver et al., 2007). Candidate mechanisms that control DNA demethylation have recently been described, including the putative DNA demethylase Growth Arrest and DNA Damage 45 Beta (*GADD45B*), as well as oxidation of methylated cytosines to 5-hydroxymethylcytosine (5hmC) followed by nucleotide excision (Hackett et al., 2013; Ma et al., 2009). In addition to its role in DNA demethylation, 5hmC is a putative epigenetic modification with the potential to regulate gene transcription (Branco, Ficz, & Reik, 2012; Mellén, Ayata, Dewell, Kriaucionis, & Heintz, 2012). This novel epigenetic modification may also be of relevance for child neurodevelopment given its enrichment in the brain (Jin, Wu, Li, & Pfeifer, 2011; Kriaucionis & Heintz, 2009), association with synaptic genes and dynamic regulation in early development (Ruzov et al., 2011; Szulwach et al., 2011), and emerging evidence of associations with psychosis (Gavin et al., 2012) and dementia (Chouliaras et al., 2013).

Collectively, these modifications alter the structure and chemical properties of the DNA and thus gene expression. As such, modifications to the DNA and its chromatin environment can be considered as an additional layer of information that is contained within the genome. Furthermore, unlike the underlying DNA sequence, which remains static across development, epigenetic modifications are dynamically regulated and responsive to changes in the environment. This is illustrated using the example of DNA methylation; however, it should be noted that chromatin modifications and histone variants (Thambirajah et al., unpublished observations) show similar dynamism across development.

7.2 DNA Methylation in Development

Until very recently, it was thought that DNA methylation patterns on the genome were overlaid only during early periods in embryonic development. Indeed, DNA methylation is considered a fundamental feature of cell differentiation. It is important to consider a simple feature of cell biology: all cells in the body generally share the same DNA. Thus the processes of cell specialization, whereby liver cells specialize in functions related to energy metabolism and brain cells establish the capacity for learning and memory, involves silencing certain regions of the genome in a manner that is specific for each cell type. Genes associated with gluconeogenesis are silenced in brain cells but remain active in liver cells. Such processes define the function of the cell type (e.g., Fan et al., 2005). DNA methylation is considered a mechanism for the genomic silencing that underlies the cell specialization of the 300 or more different cell types in the human body. Such events occur early in development and are considered to be highly stable, such that de-differentiation (whereby a cell loses its specialization) is rare and is often associated with organ dysfunction and pathologies such as cancer (Hansen et al., 2011; Irizarry et al., 2009).

7.2.1 Maternal Regulation of Stress Reactivity in the Offspring

Epigenetic modifications, such as DNA methylation, are ideal candidates to explain the lasting influence of maternal effects on offspring development. Such epigenetic modifications provide a relatively static genome with the capacity to respond to environmental challenges. Some of the first epigenetic studies to show an effect of the early environment focus on variations in maternal behavior in rats in the absence of any experimental manipulations (i.e., naturally occurring variations in mother–pup interactions). Variations of maternal care in rats are studied with simple, albeit time-consuming observations of animals in their home cages (Champagne, 2008; Champagne, Francis, Mar, & Meaney, 2003). One behavior, pup licking/grooming (LG), emerges as highly variable across mothers. Dams for which the frequency of pup LG over the first week after delivery is 1 SD > than the mean for the breeding cohort are designated as "high LG" mothers. Those for which the frequency of pup LG lies 1 SD < the mean are considered as "low LG" mothers. Such variations in the frequency of pup LG are highly stable across individual litters.

Pup LG is a major source of tactile stimulation for the neonatal rat, which regulates endocrine and cardiovascular function in the pup (Levine, 1994; Schanberg, Evoniuk, & Kuhn, 1984). The tactile stimulation derived from pup LG increases levels of growth hormone and decreases that of adrenal glucocorticoids. In line with this, the male or female adult offspring of High LG mothers show more modest behavioral and endocrine responses to stress compared to animals reared by Low LG mothers (Caldji et al., 1998; Francis, Diorio, Liu, & Meaney, 1999; Liu et al., 1997; Menard, Champagne, & Meaney, 2004; Toki et al., 2007; Weaver et al., 2004). Specifically, the offspring of High LG mothers show reduced fearfulness and more modest hypothalamic-pituitary-adrenal (HPA) responses to acute stress. Cross-fostering studies, in which pups born to High LG mothers are fostered at birth to Low LG mothers (and vice versa), reveal a direct relationship between maternal care and the postnatal development of individual differences in behavioral and HPA responses to stress (Caldji, Diorio, & Meaney, 2003; Caldji, Francis, Sharma, Plotsky, & Meaney, 2000; Francis et al., 1999; Weaver et al., 2004). In these studies, the rearing mother determined the phenotype of the offspring. Thus, variations within a normal range of parental care can dramatically alter phenotypic development in the rat.

The differences in the HPA response to stress in the offspring of High and Low LG mothers are mediated by a maternal effect on the expression of the glucocorticoid receptor gene (*Nr3c1*) in the hippocampus (Liu et al., 1997; Weaver et al., 2004, 2007). The glucocorticoid receptor is a ligand-gated nuclear receptor, which when bound by glucocorticoids is activated and translocated to the cell nucleus where it functions as a transcription factor that regulates gene expression. Glucocorticoid receptor activation in the hippocampus associates with the activation of a negative-feedback signal that regulates corticotropin-releasing factor (CRF) expression in the hypothalamus. Since CRF serves to activate the pituitary-adrenal stress response, negative-feedback regulation serves to moderate the magnitude of the stress response. The offspring of High, compared with Low, LG mothers show increased hippocampal glucocorticoid receptor expression, more efficient negative-feedback regulation of CRF, reduced hypothalamic CRF expression, and more modest HPA responses to stress.

The critical feature of the maternal effects described above is persistence. The differences in the frequency of pup LG between High and Low LG mothers are limited to the first week of postnatal life. And yet the differences in gene expression and neural function are apparent well into adulthood. These findings raise the obvious question of how an essentially social interaction stably alters the expression of the genes that regulate that activity of neural systems that mediate endocrine and behavioral responses to stress. To address this question, we focused on the sustained effect of maternal care on glucocorticoid receptor gene transcription in the hippocampus as a model system for the environmental programming of gene expression. We hypothesized that maternal licking might activate intracellular signals that would lead to a stable epigenetic state on the region of the genome that regulates glucocorticoid receptor expression, thus serving to sustain the "maternal effect" on glucocorticoid receptor expression.

The focus of the epigenetic studies with the rodent studies of maternal care is the nerve growth factor-induced protein A (NGFI-A) consensus sequence in the exon 1_7 promoter, which activates glucocorticoid receptor expression in hippocampal neurons. The tactile stimulation associated with pup LG increases serotonin (5-HT) activity in the hippocampus. In vitro studies with cultured hippocampal neurons show that 5-HT acts on 5-HT7 receptors to initiate a series of intracellular signals that culminate with an increase in the expression of NGFI-A and CREB-binding protein. Comparable effects occur in vivo. Manipulations that increase pup LG by lactating rats result in an increased level of cAMP as well as NGFI-A (Meaney et al., 2000). Pups reared by High LG mothers show increased NGFI-A expression in hippocampal neurons as well as an increased binding of NGFI-A to the exon 1_7 promoter sequence (Hellstrom, Dhir, Diorio, & Meaney, 2012; Weaver et al., 2007). Moreover, the binding of NGFI-A to the exon 1_7 promoter sequence is actively regulated by mother–pup interactions, such that there is increased NGFI-A bound to the exon 1_7 promoter immediately following a nursing bout but not at a period that follows 25 minutes without mother–pup contact (Hellstrom et al., 2012).

These findings reflect what is referred to as de novo DNA methylation, whereby a methyl group is applied to previously unmethylated sites. However, between the day following birth and the end of the first week of life, the 5' CpG is "demethylated" in pups reared by High but not Low LG mothers. This difference then persists into adulthood. Importantly, the period over which the demethylation occurs falls precisely within that time when High and Low LG mothers differ in the frequency of pup LG; the difference in pup LG between High and Low LG mothers is not apparent in the second week of postnatal life (Caldji et al., 1998; Champagne, 2008; Champagne et al., 2003).

These findings suggest that maternal licking of pups increases NGFI-A levels in the hippocampal neurons of the offspring, thus altering DNA methylation of the 5' CpG. But there is a complication. If DNA methylation blocks transcription factor binding and the 5' CpG site of the exon 1_7 promoter is heavily methylated in neonates, then how might maternally activated NGFI-A bind to and remodel the exon 1_7 region? The answer to these questions appears to involve other transcriptional signals that are affected by maternal care. Levels of the transcription factor specific protein-1 (SP-1) and the CREB-binding protein are also increased in the hippocampus of pups reared by High LG mothers (Hellstrom et al., 2012; Weaver et al., 2007). The exon 1_7 promoter contains a DNA sequence that binds SP-1, and this region overlaps with that for NGFI-A. SP-1 can actively target both methylation and demethylation of CpG sites (Brandeis et al., 1994; Macleod, Charlton, Mullins, & Bird, 1994). The 5'CpG site is the region of overlap in the binding sites. The CREB-binding protein, on the other hand, acts as a histone acetyltransferase, an enzyme capable of acetylating histone tails, including the exon 1_7 region, opening chromatin and permitting the binding of transcription factors such as NGFI-A and SP-1. Increasing histone acetylation can lead to transcription factor binding at previously methylated sites and the subsequent demethylation of these regions (Fan et al., 2005; Szyf, Weaver, Champagne, Diorio, & Meaney, 2005). Thus we suggest that the binding of this complex of proteins including NGFI-A, the CREB-binding protein, and SP-1 is critical in activating the process of demethylation. The results to date are certainly consistent with this model.

The findings discussed above suggest that maternally induced increases in hippocampal NGFI-A levels can initiate the remodeling of DNA methylation at the regions of the DNA that regulate glucocorticoid receptor expression. The NGFI-A transcription factor binds to multiple sites across the genome. If NGFI-A related complexes target demethylation, then one might assume that other NGFI-A sensitive regions should show a maternal effect on DNA methylation and gene expression comparable to that observed with the glucocorticoid receptor. Zhang et al. (2010) showed that the hippocampal expression of the *GAD1* gene that encodes for glutamic acid decarboxylase, an enzyme in the production of the neurotransmitter GABA, is increased in the adult offspring of High LG mothers. This effect is associated with altered DNA methylation of an NGFI-A response element in a manner comparable to that for the glucocorticoid receptor gene. These studies highlight perhaps the most likely candidate mechanism to explain environmental regulation of the epigenome, i.e., via transcriptional factor-mediated remodeling of DNA methylation. It should be noted that steroid receptors such the glucocorticoid, estrogen, progesterone, and estrogen receptors have the capacity to bind DNA and thus influence variation in DNA methylation.

In summary, the maternally induced changes in specific intracellular signals in hippocampal neurons can physically remodel the epigenome. The increased binding of NGFI-A that derives from pup LG appears critical for the demethylation of the exon 1_7 promoter. We suggest that this process involves accompanying increases in SP-1 and the CREB-binding protein and that the combination of these factors results in the active demethylation of the exon 1_7 promoter, a model with support from recent studies in embryonic stem cells (Lienert et al., 2011). The events described to date represent a model by which the biological pathways activated by a social event may become imprinted onto the genome. This imprint is then physically apparent in the adult genome, resulting in stable alterations (or programming) of gene expression. Similar findings have now been reported for other models of early life stress in rodents (Mueller & Bale, 2008; Murgatroyd et al., 2009) and non-human primates (Provençal et al., 2012) demonstrating lasting maternal effects on the epigenome and associated neurobehavioral phenotype of her offspring. The evidence for similar processes in humans is discussed below.

7.3 Clinical Studies of the Early Environment and DNA Methylation

A critical question is whether adversity experienced early in development in humans is linked to the stable epigenetic regulation of gene expression, as in rodents. Translational studies using human postmortem brain samples have begun to address this question. Approximately a third of individuals who die by suicide have histories of childhood adversity, including childhood sexual and physical abuse, as well as parental neglect. Labonté et al. (2012) and McGowan et al. (2009) showed decreased hippocampal GR expression in samples from suicide completers with histories of childhood maltreatment compared with controls (sudden, involuntary fatalities). Psychological autopsies (forensic interviews with family members) have been used to establish the developmental history and mental health status of suicide completers (Dumais et al., 2005; Zouk, Tousignant, Seguin, Lesage, & Turecki, 2006). McGowan et al. (2009) found no association between a history of mood disorders or substance use and hippocampal GR expression. Rather, decreased hippocampal GR expression was associated with a history of childhood maltreatment. In fact, there were no differences in hippocampal GR expression in samples from suicides negative for a history of childhood maltreatment. Instead, the differences in hippocampal GR expression were unique to suicide completers with a history of childhood maltreatment.

Splice variant analysis, comparable to that performed in rats, revealed decreased expression of non-coding exons 1_B, 1_C, 1_F, and 1_H in suicides with a history of childhood maltreatment compared with both controls and suicides without a history of maltreatment. These expression differences correlated with differential DNA methylation patterns between groups in the corresponding exon 1 variant promoters. The exon 1_F sequence is of particular interest as it is the homolog of the rat exon 1_7, is highly expressed in brain, and contains an NGFI-A response element (McGowan et al., 2009; Turner & Muller, 2005). Moreover, the exon 1_F sequence shows increased DNA methylation and decreased NGFI-A binding in samples from suicide completers with a history of maltreatment. These findings bear considerable similarity to the maternal effect in rats and are suggestive of early-environment regulation of the neural epigenome in humans. Studies in independent human samples investigating the effects of early-environmental adversity on exon 1_F methylation reported consistent results (Radtke et al., 2011; Tyrka, Price, Marsit, Walters, & Carpenter, 2012 and see below), with a recent systematic review concluding that 89% of human studies and 70% of animal studies were directionally consistent with early adversity predicting increased DNA methylation of the glucocorticoid receptor (Turecki & Meaney, 2014).

The English and Romanian Adoptees (ERA) study (Rutter et al., 2012; Sonuga-Barke et al., 2017) and the Bucharest Early Intervention Project (BEIP) highlight the profound influence of the early care environment on child neurodevelopment and vulnerability for mental disorders (McGoron et al., 2012; Nelson et al., 2007; O'Connor, Rutter, Beckett, Keaveney, & Kreppner, 2000; Rutter et al., 2012; Sheridan, Fox, Zeanah, McLaughlin, & Nelson, 2012). Such cohorts are fertile ground for epigenetic studies. Kumsta et al. (2016) find some evidence to suggest early institutionalization influences variation in the DNA methylome. The authors identify a differentially methylation region (DMR) in *CYP2E1* in adolescents (15 years of age) with a history of extended institutionalization (>6 months; $n = 16$) relative to individuals who were institutionalized for <6 months. DNA methylation of this region is also associated with aspects of IQ and social cognition (Kumsta et al., 2016). Conversely, Non et al. (2016) adopt a more targeted approach and report associations between history of institutionalization and DNA methylation of

SLC6A4 and *FKBP5* in adolescents from the BEIP ($n = 117$; $n = 82$ ever institutionalized and $n = 35$ never institutionalized). Findings from Grigorenko and colleagues indicate that such children deprived of parental care show distinct epigenetic changes at least into adolescence (Naumova et al., 2016). Naumova et al. (2012) assessed the methylation status of approximately 27,000 CpGs in 14 children raised in federal institutions and 14 controls, ranging between 8 and 14 years of age (Naumova et al., 2012). The authors observed that 3.5% of CpG sites show evidence of differential methylation. A shift towards hypermethylation of target genes associated with immune response and cellular signaling was observed in the institutionalized group. The functional effects of these epigenetic changes on vulnerability for psychopathology have not been reported; however, this study provides proof of principle that the absence of parental care influences DNA methylation in humans.

Additional genome-wide analyses of DNA methylation reveal the pervasive effect of early adversity on the methylome (Essex et al., 2013; Labonté et al., 2012; Mehta et al., 2013; Yang et al., 2013). Turecki and colleagues characterized the effects of childhood abuse on DNA methylation using adult hippocampal samples (Labonté et al., 2012) and reported differential methylation of 362 gene promoters in hippocampal neurons associated with cellular/neuronal plasticity. Yang et al. (2013) reported a greater number of differentially methylated targets (2868) affected by childhood abuse; however, this analysis was conducted closer in time to the exposure and used a mixed cell population from saliva. Similarly, maternal stress, especially early in infancy, is predictive of DNA methylation profiles assessed in buccal epithelial cells at age 15 years (Essex et al., 2013). More recently, Mehta et al. (2013) showed that childhood adversity associates with coordinated epigenetic and transcriptional changes in peripheral blood cells from adults with PTSD (Mehta et al., 2013). Interestingly, despite a similar clinical presentation for both groups (i.e., PTSD), early life adversity was associated with an almost unique transcriptional profile relative to PTSD patients without early life exposure, suggesting differential regulation of gene transcription in this group. These cross-sectional analyses of children with a history of institutionalization provide proof of principle of the effect of early social deprivation on variation in DNA methylation. Future studies will be required to determine if these changes in DNA methylation are predictive of adult psychopathology.

Collectively, these studies suggest that the early social environment influences epigenetic mechanisms in both neural tissue and peripheral sources. A question remains about the functional importance of these changes, which will need to be addressed with appropriate in vitro models examining individual sites. Moreover, the statistical models used to detect "affected" CpGs remain an issue of some debate, and existing reports of the actual number of differentially methylated CpG sites should be considered as estimates. For example, the Illumina MethylationEPIC Beadchip (850 K array), currently considered the gold standard for large-scale epigenetic epidemiology, surveys less than 4% of the human DNA methylome. As such, the number of CpGs associated with a phenotype of interest is likely to vary as a function of the amount of the DNA methylome assessed. Perhaps a greater concern is the degree to which DNA methylation profiles established in peripheral sources of DNA are informative about epigenetic mechanisms within the brain (see Table 7.1).

Table 7.1 Overview of studies on early adversity and epigenetics with a GWAS approach

Authors (years)	Title	Methods	*N*	Exposure	Main findings
Cicchetti, Hetzel, Rogosch, Handley, and Toth (2016)	An investigation of child maltreatment and epigenetic mechanisms of mental and physical health risk	HumanMethylation450 BeadChip (Illumina)	548	Low SES 54.4% of the sample had a history of childhood maltreatment	Girls who experienced maltreatment presented with significantly lower methylation for ALDH2 than non-maltreated girls. Higher methylation levels were also found in maltreated boys compared to the non-maltreated ones Significantly higher methylation for ALDH2 was found in early onset—not recently maltreated boys compared to non-maltreated boys. The same finding was found in children with early onset—Non-recent maltreatment compared to non-maltreated children at ANKK1 Maltreated children presented with different methylation levels for several disease indices compared to non-maltreated children When high levels of methylation at CpG sites were observed in maltreated children, non-maltreated children presented with low and medium levels of methylation. In addition, maltreated children methylation levels were found to be low at CpG sites where non-maltreated children's methylation levels were high
Mehta et al. (2013)	Childhood maltreatment is associated with distinct genomic and epigenetic profiles in posttraumatic stress disorder	Human methylation 450 k BeadChip (Illumina)	169	Childhood adversity	Results showed that in adults suffering from PTSD, childhood adversity was correlated with coordinated epigenetic and transcriptional changes in peripheral blood cells

Yang et al. (2013)	Child abuse and epigenetic mechanisms of disease risk	Illumina 450 K methylation BeadChip	192	Maltreatment	Methylation levels were significantly different in maltreated children and controls at 2868 CpG sites Markers of diseases and biological processes related to health problems found after exposure to early childhood adversity were found in those genes
Labonté et al. (2012)	Genome-wide epigenetic regulation by early life trauma	meDIP, 400 K (custom)	41	Abused, suicide	Individuals with a history of abuse had 362 differentially methylated promoters compared with controls 248 of those promoters presented hypermethylation, whereas 114 were hypomethylated
Naumova et al. (2012)	Differential patterns of whole-genome DNA methylation in institutionalized children and children raised by their biological parents	Infinium HumanMethylation27 BeadChip array	28	Institutionalization	Institutionalized children presented with higher methylation levels compared to the control group, for most part in genes implicated in the control of immune response and cellular signaling systems

7.4 Tissue Specificity: DNA Methylation in the Blood and Brain

As discussed above, DNA methylation is, in part, responsible for cell-fate specification. As such, DNA methylation is tissue and indeed cell-type specific (Deaton et al., 2011; Rakyan et al., 2008; Varley et al., 2013). This specificity poses a challenge to researchers studying DNA methylation in the context of child psychiatry where access to neural tissue is unavailable. A number of recent studies have addressed this issue by comparing DNA methylation profiles in both the blood and brain (Davies et al., 2012; Edgar, Jones, Robinson, & Kobor, 2017; Farre et al., 2015; Provençal et al., 2012; Ursini et al., 2011).

Ursini et al. (2011) reported findings from a clinical sample in which an interaction between stressful life events and Catechol-*o*-methyltransferase genotype predicted *COMT* methylation in peripheral blood and working memory performance during an fMRI task. The authors used adult rat prefrontal cortex and blood samples to demonstrate a moderate correlation between *COMT* methylation across tissues ($r = 0.50$); however, the degree of association in human samples is unknown. This study used a very appropriate approach, as the correspondence between methylation states in the brain and peripheral tissues is likely to vary as a function of genomic region. Such a focus on candidate genes is a valuable compliment to studies using genome-wide assessment.

Provençal et al. (2012) use a genome-wide approach to describe the long-term effects of the early rearing environment on DNA methylation in the blood and brain of adult rhesus macaques. Maternal versus peer rearing, a manipulation that leads to persistent and marked changes in behavior and stress reactivity, associates with differential methylation of 1981 probes in the prefrontal cortex but only 227 sites in a selected peripheral T cell population. A weak correlation was observed between differentially methylated probes between the two tissues ($r = 0.07$). It should be noted that this study focused exclusively on gene promoter methylation. In humans, Davies et al. (2012) provide a comprehensive description of DNA methylation in six cortical regions, the cerebellum, and matched peripheral whole blood samples. In their findings, DNA methylation within each brain region clustered together and was clearly distinct from blood. Remarkably, between-individual differences in DNA methylation identified in blood were moderately correlated with between-individual differences in brain samples ($r = 0.66$–0.76). This study contrasts with the findings of Provençal et al. (2012), which examined direct correlations of absolute methylation levels across tissues rather than between-individual differences across tissues. Collectively, these studies suggest that peripheral sources of DNA may be somewhat informative for identifying individual differences in DNA methylation of relevance to neural processes. However, an important caveat to the Davies et al. (2012) study, and to genome-wide analyses in general, is that large regions of the genome (e.g., retrotransposons) should be highly methylated regardless of cell type. The inclusion of such regions into analyses is likely to inflate the degree of correspondence across cell types.

More recently, Edgar, Jones, Meaney, Turecki, and Kobor (2017) have established a blood-brain DNA methylome resource, which facilitates a direct comparison of the cross-tissue concordance of DNA methylation levels in blood and brain (Edgar, Jones, Meaney, et al., 2017). The Blood-Brain Epigenetic Concordance tool provides variance and concordance estimates across ~450,000 CpG sites contained on the Illumina humanmethylation450 (450 K array) using data from 16 individuals with paired blood and brain samples. Such resources, using a wider range of peripheral tissues, will be required to address issues of cross-tissue concordance for early life adversity effects on DNA methylation.

In addition to questions regarding tissue specificity, an increasing number of studies assess the stability of DNA methylation over time. This issue is critical for studies examining the potential of DNA methylation marks to serve as biomarkers for later psychopathology. The role of DNA methylation in developmental processes such as X-inactivation, genomic imprinting, and tissue differentiation suggests that DNA methylation is a highly stable epigenetic modification. Nevertheless, at certain sites DNA methylation can be dynamic (e.g., Herb et al., 2012; Lister et al., 2013; Martinowich et al., 2003; Nelson, Kavalali, & Monteggia, 2008). Cross-sectional, longitudinal, and twin studies now describe variation in DNA methylation across development. A study in newborns and centenarians reports more widespread hypomethylation and greater variability in DNA methylation between CpG sites in the elderly relative to the more uniformly methylated newborn DNA (Heyn et al., 2012). Similarly, Fraga et al. (2005) show increasing epigenetic discordance in monozygotic twins across ages. However, discordance in DNA methylation between monozygotic twins exists even at birth, suggesting intrauterine effects (Gordon et al., 2012; and see Kaminsky et al., 2009). Indeed, rates of change may not be linear across the lifespan, with studies suggesting more dynamic change between 3 and 17 years (Alisch et al., 2012). Two longitudinal studies examine the stability of DNA methylation in infancy. Wang et al. (2012) examined DNA methylation at approximately 27,000 CpGs in cord and venous blood samples at birth and the first 24 months of life (average follow-up was 12 months of age). The authors found remarkable stability over time with significant changes occurring at <1% of probes assessed (Wang et al., 2012). In contrast, Martino et al. (2011) show more dynamic change in mononuclear DNA methylation in their study of 0–5-year-olds. DNA methylation profiles from female newborns and 1- and 5-year-olds tended to form distinct clusters, while the 2.5-year-old group clustered with both 1- and 5-year-olds. Such individual differences in DNA methylation in the postnatal period may point to differential susceptibility of certain individuals to environmental factors that influence DNA methylation (Martino et al., 2011). Moreover, there is also very likely to be variation in the stability of DNA methylation as a function of cell type, with perhaps the more phenotypically variable cells associated with immune function showing greater variation than those in other cell types. In a more recent study, Martino et al. (2013) examined longitudinal changes in DNA methylation of buccal epithelial cells in monozygotic twins using the 450 K array. The authors observed an interesting pattern of twin-twin discordance that varied as a function of obstetric outcomes (e.g., birth weight). Interestingly, while some twin pairs showed a trend towards increasing concordance over time, some twin pairs showed increasing discordance across the first 18 months of life, suggesting a differential effect of the early environment on DNA methylome maturation across twin pairs. The clinical relevance of such findings is unknown; however, it is of interest that despite a largely similar genetic background, these twins showed differences in the rate of change in DNA methylation at specific sites.

The finding that DNA methylation changes over time and across age groups has led to the development of epigenetic predictors of chronological age. The "epigenetic clock" derived from DNA methylation of 353 CpGs (Horvath, 2013) has emerged as a cross-tissue index of biological aging. Epigenetic age acceleration (Δage) (chronological minus epigenetic age) represents a feature of the DNA methylome associated with cumulative lifetime stress (Zannas et al., 2015) and is predictive of cognitive fitness, mortality, and a range of health outcomes across multiple cohorts (Chen et al., 2016; Horvath et al., 2012; Marioni et al., 2015). Δage predicts adverse health outcomes often comorbid with exposure to early life adversity and is increased by lifetime stress exposure (Zannas et al., 2015). This effect of stress on Δage is mediated by glucocorticoid (GC) remodeling of DNA methylation at GC-sensitive clock CpGs (Zannas et al., 2015). Notably, dysregulated GC signaling is often associated with exposure to early adversity, including child maltreatment (Heim et al., 2001; Trickett, Noll, Susman, Shenk, & Putnam, 2010), suggesting Δage might be a useful indicator of sensitivity to early life adversity. However, no study to date has examined the association between Δage and common mental disorders such as major depressive disorder, which often covary with exposure to early adversity. This seems like a logical avenue for exploration, especially in light of the findings of Brody, Yu, Chen, Beach, and Miller (2015), who showed that a psychosocial parenting intervention moderates the effects of parental depression on Δage in adolescent offspring. Similar analyses within the context of intervention programs that reduce rates of child maltreatment or mitigate some of the adverse effects of exposure to maltreatment are lacking. Such evidence is required to evaluate the utility of the DNA methylome for personalized approaches in the fields of perinatal psychiatry and child/adolescent mental health.

Likewise, a limitation of the current epigenetic clock is the prediction error within epigenetic age estimates (~3.6 years). Such a large error may limit the interpretation of age estimates in pediatric cohorts and in cohorts with a narrow age range. Current efforts to develop a pediatric epigenetic clock (McEwen et al., personal communication) may prove more informative for studies in maltreated youth. Finally, a recent study has examined the heritability of Δage (Lu et al., 2016). Intriguingly, heritability demonstrated tissue specificity, which suggests that both genetic and environmental influences on epigenetic aging may differentially affect different tissues. This finding further highlights the need to consider genetic variation even in studies that use broad indices of the DNA methylome such as the epigenetic clock.

7.5 The Importance of Genotype in Studies of the Epigenome

Data from twin and multigenerational studies suggest a genetic influence on epigenetic modifications such as DNA methylation (Gertz et al., 2011; Kaminsky et al., 2009; Zhang et al., 2010). Indeed, an exciting area of current (and future) investigation research in psychiatric (epi)genetics is the integration of genetic and epigenetic data with relevant measures of the early environment.

Genetic polymorphism and epigenetic modifications both influence gene transcription. It is important to emphasize that these are coordinated and often interdependent processes. For example, 5-methylcytosine is more readily mutated to thymine, leading to mismatched guanine-thymine pairs, which are further modified to create an A-T bond. This process may, in part, explain the reduced frequency of CpGs across the human genome (Deaton & Bird, 2011). Similarly, genotype is an important determinant of the epigenetic landscape (Lienert et al., 2011). A recent analysis of DNA methylation in six individuals from a three-generation family illustrates that DNA methylation reflects genetic relatedness (Gertz et al., 2011). Gertz et al. (2011) reported that genotype may account for 80% of the variance in DNA methylation, finding many of the allele-specific effects identified in the related individuals were also seen in unrelated individuals. Similarly, widespread effects of genotype on DNA methylation in the human brain have been reported (Zhang, Cheng, et al., 2010) with some evidence that genotype-methylation associations are conserved across peripheral and neural tissues (Docherty et al., 2012; Klengel et al., 2013), permitting the study of such associations in peripheral tissue.

Genotype may influence DNA methylation in a number of ways. Genetic polymorphisms (SNPs, VNTRs, CNVs) may introduce or remove CpGs, thereby adding (or removing) potential sites for methylation. Genetic polymorphisms that modulate transcription factor binding may also influence DNA methylation events. Increased transcription factor binding can protect CpG islands from DNA methylation and vice versa (Lienert et al., 2011; Macleod et al., 1994; Stadler et al., 2011). Both gene promoter and more distal regulatory regions appear to be influenced by transcription factor binding in this way (Schubeler, 2012). Genotypic variation may also act in *trans* to influence activity cell signaling pathways that trigger changes in DNA methylation (Bonder et al., 2017). Collectively, these findings point to a strong association between genotype and DNA methylation. Furthermore, there is emerging evidence that such genotype-methylation interdependency may be influenced by the early environment (Klengel et al., 2013; Ursini et al., 2011; Vijayendran, Beach, Plume, Brody, & Philibert, 2012). These allele-specific effects provide a biological mechanism to explain statistical G × E associations.

The concept of G × E effects on vulnerability for mental disorder has been a major paradigm shift in child psychiatry (Caspi & Moffitt, 2006; Meaney, 2010). Initial reports demonstrated that environmental factors such as childhood maltreatment (Caspi et al., 2002), stressful life events (Caspi et al., 2003), and cannabis use (Caspi et al., 2005) interact with genetic risk factors to predict risk of later mental disorder. These reports have been supported and extended by clinical and basic research over the past 15 years (Meaney, 2010; however see Risch et al., 2009; but also Rutter, Thapar, & Pickles, 2009). More recently, G × E effects have been reported that provide support for the parent-signaling hypothesis. For example, children carrying the dopamine receptor D4 (DRD4) 7-repeat allele show significantly better neurodevelopmental outcomes but only when exposed to high maternal sensitivity or an enriched early care environment (Belsky & Pluess, 2013; Berry, Deater-Deckard, McCartney, Wang, & Petrill, 2013). Indeed, the presence of the DRD4 7-repeat allele was associated with increased risk of adverse outcomes in children exposed to low maternal sensitivity and poor early care.

Despite an increased appreciation for the importance and biological plausibility of G × E effects, the molecular basis for these associations remains poorly defined. Epigenetic modifications, such as DNA methylation, provide a mechanism to link genetic and environmental risk to phenotype (Klengel et al., 2013; Meaney, 2010). In addition to our work in rats, two recent human studies provide evidence for a molecular definition of G × E effects. The first, drawn from the Iowa adoption study (Beach, Brody, Todorov, Gunter, & Philibert, 2010), demonstrates that exposure to childhood sexual abuse and being a carrier of the short version of the *SLC6A4* repeat polymorphism interact to predict decreased methylation of a CpG within *SLC6A4*. While this study, which used immortalized cell lines, failed to find an association between this interaction term and *SLC6A4* mRNA levels, it did provide proof of principle for G × E influences on epigenetic marks. More recently, Klengel et al. (2013) provided a comprehensive description of allele-specific demethylation of the glucocorticoid receptor co-regulator *FKBP5* in adults exposed to childhood trauma. This study demonstrated that polymorphisms in *FKBP5* influence the position of the nucleosome, which when combined with childhood trauma (postulated to increase circulating cortisol) results in increased risk of PTSD. At the molecular level, this interaction is associated with stable DNA demethylation, increased transcription of *FKBP5*, symptoms of glucocorticoid resistance, and reduced hippocampal volume. In line with what is known about the capacity for transcription factors to modulate local DNA methylation levels, a large emphasis is placed on the presence of a glucocorticoid response element, which may be an important mediator of these demethylation events (Klengel et al., 2013). Ursini et al. (2011) also provide evidence that environmental stress and genotype may interact to produce allele-specific changes in DNA methylation, which are in turn associated with cognitive performance. In summary, these studies build on epidemiological analyses of G × E effects by providing a functional mechanism to link genetic risk factors and adverse environmental exposures to sustained physiological changes relevant to mental health. Undoubtedly, both candidate gene and genome-wide analyses will uncover additional genomic regions with epigenetic modification in response to early adversity (see Table 7.2).

Table 7.2 Overview of studies on early adversity and epigenetics with a candidate gene approach

Authors (years)	Title	Methods	*N*	Exposure	Locus	Main findings
Hecker, Radtke, Hermenau, Papassotiropoulos, and Elbert (2016)	Associations among child abuse, mental health, and epigenetic modifications in the proopiomelanocortin gene (POMC): A study with children in Tanzania	Bisulfite conversion	35 children with high abuse exposure and 35 with low exposure	Abuse	POMC	Children in the high abuse exposure group showed increased POMC DNA methylation
Kumsta et al. (2016)	Severe psychosocial deprivation in early childhood is associated with increased DNA methylation across a region spanning the transcription start site of CYP2E1	Bisulfite conversion	49	Institutionalization	Cytochrome P450 2E1 gene (CYP2E1) on chromosome 10	Children exposed to extreme early institutional deprivation showed increased DNA methylation in a region of the CYP2E1 gene
Non et al. (2016)	DNA methylation at stress-related genes is associated with exposure to early life institutionalization	Pyrosequencing	117	Institutionalization	FKBP5 SLC6A4	Children who spent more time in institutional care showed reduced DNA methylation at specific CpG sites within both FKBP5 and SLC6A4 genes
Tyrka, Ridout, and Parade (2016)	Methylation of the leukocyte glucocorticoid receptor gene promoter in adults: Associations with early adversity and depressive, anxiety and substance-use disorders	EZ DNA methylation kit	340	Childhood maltreatment	Exon 1F of NR3C1	Exposure to childhood maltreatment was associated with reduced methylation of NR3C1

(continued)

Table 7.2 (continued)

Authors (years)	Title	Methods	*N*	Exposure	Locus	Main findings
Yehuda et al. (2016)	Holocaust exposure induced intergenerational effects on FKBP5 methylation	Sodium bisulfite pyrosequencing	40	Holocaust exposure	FKBP5	Holocaust survivors had increased methylation at bin 3/site6 of FKBP5 Contrastingly, offspring of holocaust survivors showed decreased methylation at bin 3/site6 of FKBP5
Tyrka et al. (2015)	Childhood maltreatment and methylation of FK506 binding protein 5 gene (FKBP5)	Sodium bisulfite pyrosequencing	174	Childhood maltreatment and trauma	FKBP5	Children with a history of maltreatment showed decreased FKBP5 methylation at CpGs 1 and 2 A composite score of trauma and maltreatment experiences was associated with decreased methylation of FKBP5 at CpG1
Yehuda et al. (2015)	Lower methylation of glucocorticoid receptor gene promoter 1F in peripheral blood of veterans with posttraumatic stress disorder	Bisulfite conversion	122	PTSD	NR3C1	Combat veterans with PTSD showed decreased NR3C1-1F promoter methylation in peripheral blood mononuclear cells (PBMCs) as compared to veterans without PTSD
Perroud et al. (2014)	The Tutsi genocide and transgenerational transmission of maternal stress: Epigenetics and biology of the HPA axis	Pyrosequencing	25	PTSD	NR3C1 NR3C2	Mothers that were exposed to the Tutsi genocide and their children showed increased methylation of the NR3C1 exon 1_F compared to the non-exposed group. Exposed mothers also had increased methylation of CpGs located within the NR3C2 coding sequence vs. non-exposed mothers

Yehuda et al. (2014)	Influences of maternal and paternal PTSD on epigenetic regulation of the glucocorticoid receptor gene in holocaust survivor offspring	Bisulfite conversion	122	Maternal and paternal PTSD	GR-1_F	Children whose fathers had PTSD showed increased GR-1^F promoter methylation Contrastingly, children for whose both parents had PTSD showed decreased methylation
Klengel et al. (2013)	Allele-specific bp5 DNA demethylation mediates gene-childhood trauma interactions	Sodium bisulfite pyrosequencing	129?	Childhood trauma	FKBP5	Childhood trauma was associated with FKBP5 demethylation but only for risk allele carriers

7.6 Methodological Considerations for Studies of Epigenetics in Child Psychiatry

The importance of epigenetics for studies of maltreated youth is emphasized by a recent wave of epigenome-wide association studies. These analyses are beginning to uncover disease-risk markers in peripheral tissue for conditions often associated with exposure to early adversity, such as schizophrenia and bipolar disorder (Dempster et al., 2011; Hannon et al., 2016), major depression (Byrne et al., 2013; Sabunciyan et al., 2012), posttraumatic stress disorder (Mehta et al., 2013; Smith et al., 2011), and autism (Berko et al., 2014; Wong et al., 2013). A critical question in the field of epigenetic epidemiology is the choice of tissue for such studies. For studies of neurodevelopment and mental health, an argument has been made in support of saliva (Smith et al., 2015) or buccal epithelial cells (Berko et al., 2014; Kumsta et al., 2016). This is largely due to brain and buccal cells sharing the same lineage, i.e., arising from the ectoderm. There is some suggestive evidence in support of this argument; however, a definitive study is required (Isagawa, Wang, Kobayashi, Itoh, & Maeda, 2011; Papavassiliou et al., 2009).

A related issue in such studies is the issue of cellular heterogeneity (Lappalainen & Greally, 2017). While methods exist to statistically predict the proportion of major cell types in blood and buccal samples from DNA methylation data, such reference-based methods do not fully capture the diversity of cell types that exist in these biosamples. Indeed, this issue of confounding by cell type has been identified previously where cell type has been shown to inflate the number of CpGs associated with disease status (Liu et al., 2013), early institutionalization (Esposito et al., 2016), or SES experienced in early life (Lam et al., 2012). The question arises as to how the early environment influences the proportion of cells in a given biosample to give rise to such confounding effects.

Several of the EWAS studies described above employed microarray-based platforms for methylation analyses. Currently, the 850 K array provides the most comprehensive genome-wide coverage (>850,000 CpG and non-CG sites) at a cost that permits its use in larger scale, epidemiological-like studies. It should be noted that despite improved genome-wide coverage, this array provides quantitative data on >4% of the 28 million CpGs contained in the human genome. An advantage of the 850 K array is that it includes increased coverage of enhancer sites, which are gaining increased prominence in studies of environmental regulation of the genome (Pidsley et al., 2016). Next-generation sequencing approaches to methylation analyses such as reduced representation of bisulfite sequencing and whole-genome bisulfite sequencing may reveal novel genomic regions of interest, sensitive to maternal effects and relevant for child vulnerability for mental disorder; however, the cost of such sequencing to resolve relatively small differences in DNA methylation may be prohibitively expensive for large epidemiological studies (Teh et al., 2016).

An additional consideration for future studies is the need to distinguish DNA methylation (5mC) from hydroxymethylation (5hmC). Currently, studies that employ standard bisulfite conversion protocols fail to discriminate between these two different epigenetic modifications. Oxidative bisulfite sequencing is promising in this respect (Booth et al., 2012). Finally, as noted above, epigenetic modifications do not occur in isolation, nor are they independent of the underlying DNA sequence. Several in vitro studies have carried out genome-wide surveys of multiple epigenetic modifications (DNA methylation, histone posttranslational modifications and non-coding RNAs) and reveal coordinated epigenetic control of gene transcription and interactions with genotypes (Lienert et al., 2011; Reddy et al., 2012; Stadler et al., 2011) as well as evidence of cross-species conservation of specific features of the epigenome (Xiao et al., 2012). Such combined approaches may prove useful in clinical studies of early adversity and may help determine if maternal effects associated with increased risk of mental health problems are also associated with dysregulation in the coordinated epigenetic control of gene expression.

7.7 Epigenetics and Clinical Practice

Genome-wide DNA methylation (the DNA methylome) is dynamic across development (Horvath, 2013; Ziller et al., 2013) and is altered by early social experience (Lam et al., 2012; McGowan et al., 2009).

Nonetheless, challenges remain before measure of the DNA methylome can be translated to improve clinical practice. As discussed above, the choice of tissue for studies of the impact of the early environment on child neurodevelopment is yet to be established. Likewise, while DNA methylation is relatively stable, detailed longitudinal analyses are required to establish normal rates of DNA methylome maturation. Such studies would provide a better understanding of methylome dynamics as a function of development. Such data would also be required to better interpret early adversity effects on DNA methylation and whether such changes are associated with accelerated or delayed DNA methylome maturation. Prospectively designed cohorts, incorporating longitudinal biosampling, will clarify the relationship between early life adversity, the DNA methylome, and its predictive value for mental health outcomes.

7.8 Conclusions

It is clear that early life adversity, such as a history of child maltreatment, predicts a range of negative developmental outcomes, including an increased vulnerability for later mental disorders. There is emerging evidence in support of an environmental epigenetics hypothesis, with evidence that early life adversity associates with variation in epigenetic modifications such as DNA methylation. However, a question remains as to whether such effects arise as a function of changes in cell phenotype. Likewise, the evidence that such epigenetic changes mediate the effects of early life adversity on child outcomes is rather limited and requires further in-depth study.

Such efforts represent the logical next steps in advancing epigenetically informed approaches to personalized medicine. Thus, while epigenetics is an exciting and rapidly growing field, translating basic scientific findings to improve clinical care and mental health outcomes will require continued and cautious research efforts.

References

Alisch, R. S., Barwick, B. G., Chopra, P., Myrick, L. K., Satten, G. A., Conneely, K. N., & Warren, S. T. (2012). Age-associated DNA methylation in pediatric populations. *Genome Research, 22*, 623–632. https://doi.org/10.1101/gr.125187.111

Beach, S. R. H., Brody, G. H., Todorov, A. A., Gunter, T. D., & Philibert, R. A. (2010). Methylation at SLC6A4 is linked to family history of child abuse: An examination of the Iowa adoptee sample. *American Journal of Medical Genetics Part B: Neuropsychiatric Genetics, 153B*, 710–713.

Belsky, J., & Pluess, M. (2013). Genetic moderation of early child-care effects on social functioning across childhood: A developmental analysis. *Child Development, 84*, 1209–1225. https://doi.org/10.1111/cdev.12058

Berko, E. R., Suzuki, M., Beren, F., Lemetre, C., Alaimo, C. M., Calder, R. B., ... Greally, J. M. (2014). Mosaic epigenetic dysregulation of ectodermal cells in autism spectrum disorder. *PLoS Genetics, 10*, e1004402. https://doi.org/10.1371/journal.pgen.1004402PGENETICS-D-13-02792. [pii].

Berry, D., Deater-Deckard, K., McCartney, K., Wang, Z., & Petrill, S. A. (2013). Gene-environment interaction between dopamine receptor D4 7-repeat polymorphism and early maternal sensitivity predicts inattention trajectories across middle childhood. *Development and Psychopathology, 25*, 291–306. https://doi.org/10.1017/S095457941200106X. S095457941200106X [pii].

Bird, A. P. (1986). CpG-rich islands and the function of DNA methylation. *Nature, 321*, 209–213.

Bird, A. P. (2002). DNA methylation patterns and epigenetic memory. *Genes and Development, 16*, 6–21.

Bonder, M. J., Luijk, R., Zhernakova, D. V., Moed, M., Deelen, P., Vermaat, M., ... Heijmans, B. T. (2017). Disease variants alter transcription factor levels and methylation of their binding sites. *Nature Genetics, 49*, 131–138. https://doi.org/10.1038/ng.3721

Booth, M. J., Branco, M. R., Ficz, G., Oxley, D., Krueger, F., Reik, W., & Balasubramanian, S. (2012). Quantitative sequencing of 5-methylcytosine and 5-hydroxymethylcytosine at single-base resolution. *Science, 336*, 934–937. https://doi.org/10.1126/science.1220671

Branco, M. R., Ficz, G., & Reik, W. (2012). Uncovering the role of 5-hydroxymethylcytosine in the epigenome. *Nature Reviews Genetics, 13*, 7–13.

Brandeis, M., Frank, D., Keshet, I., Siegfried, Z., Mendelsohn, M., Names, A., ... Cedar, H. (1994). Spl elements protect a CpG island from de novo methylation. *Nature, 371*, 435–438.

Brody, G. H., Yu, T., Chen, E., Beach, S. R., & Miller, G. E. (2015). Family-centered prevention ameliorates the longitudinal association between risky family processes and epigenetic aging. *Journal of Child Psychology and Psychiatry, 57*, 566. https://doi.org/10.1111/jcpp.12495

Byrne, E. M., Carrillo-Roa, T., Henders, A. K., Bowdler, L., McRae, A. F., Heath, A. C., ... Wray, N. R. (2013). Monozygotic twins affected with major depressive disorder have greater variance in methylation than their unaffected co-twin. *Translational Psychiatry, 3*, e269. https://doi.org/10.1038/tp.2013.45

Caldji, C., Diorio, J., & Meaney, M. J. (2003). Variations in maternal care alter GABAA receptor subunit expression in brain regions associated with fear. *Neuropsychopharmacology, 28*, 1950–1959.

Caldji, C., Francis, D., Sharma, S., Plotsky, P. M., & Meaney, M. J. (2000). The effects of early rearing environment on the development of GABAA and central benzodiazepine receptor levels and novelty-induced fearfulness in the rat. *Neuropsychopharmacology, 22*, 219–229.

Caldji, C., Tannenbaum, B., Sharma, S., Francis, D., Plotsky, P. M., & Meaney, M. J. (1998). Maternal care during infancy regulates the development of neural systems mediating the expression of fearfulness in the rat. *Proceedings of the National Academy of Sciences of the United States of America, 95*, 5335–5340.

Caspi, A., Harrington, H., Milne, B., Amell, J. W., Theodore, R. F., & Moffitt, T. E. (2003). Children's behavioral styles at age 3 are linked to their adult personality traits at age 26. *Journal of Personality, 71*, 495–513.

Caspi, A., McClay, J., Moffitt, T. E., Mill, J., Martin, J., Craig, I. W., … Poulton, R. (2002). Role of genotype in the cycle of violence in maltreated children. *Science, 297*, 851–854. https://doi.org/10.1126/science.1072290

Caspi, A., & Moffitt, T. E. (2006). Gene-environment interactions in psychiatry: Joining forces with neuroscience. *Nature Reviews Neuroscience, 7*, 583.

Caspi, A., Moffitt, T. E., Cannon, M., McClay, J., Murray, R., Harrington, H., … Craig, I. W. (2005). Moderation of the effect of adolescent-onset cannabis use on adult psychosis by a functional polymorphism in the catechol-O-methyltransferase gene: Longitudinal evidence of a gene X environment interaction. *Biological Psychiatry, 57*, 1117–1127. S0006–3223(05)00103–4 [pii]. https://doi.org/10.1016/j.biopsych.2005.01.026

Champagne, F. A. (2008). Epigenetic mechanisms and the transgenerational effects of maternal care. *Frontiers in Neuroendocrinology, 29*, 386–397. https://doi.org/10.1016/j.yfrne.2008.03.003

Champagne, F. A., Francis, D. D., Mar, A., & Meaney, M. J. (2003). Variations in maternal care in the rat as a mediating influence for the effects of environment on development. *Physiology and Behavior, 79*, 359–371. https://doi.org/10.1016/S0031-9384(03)00149-5

Chen, B. H., Marioni, R. E., Colicino, E., Peters, M. J., Ward-Caviness, C. K., Tsai, P. C., … Horvath, S. (2016). DNA methylation-based measures of biological age: Meta-analysis predicting time to death. *Aging, 8*, 1844–1865. https://doi.org/10.18632/aging.101020

Chouliaras, L., Mastroeni, D., Delvaux, E., Grover, A., Kenis, G., Hof, P. R., … van den Hove, D. L. A. (2013). Consistent decrease in global DNA methylation and hydroxymethylation in the hippocampus of Alzheimer's disease patients. *Neurobiology of Aging, 34*, 2091. https://doi.org/10.1016/j.neurobiolaging.2013.02.021

Cicchetti, D., Hetzel, S., Rogosch, F. A., Handley, E. D., & Toth, S. L. (2016). An investigation of child maltreatment and epigenetic mechanisms of mental and physical health risk. *Development and Psychopathology, 28*, 1305–1317.

Davies, M. N., Volta, M., Pidsley, R., Lunnon, K., Dixit, A., Lovestone, S., … Mill, J. (2012). Functional annotation of the human brain methylome identifies tissue-specific epigenetic variation across brain and blood. *Genome Biology, 13*, R43. https://doi.org/10.1186/gb-2012-13-6-r43

Deaton, A. M., & Bird, A. (2011). CpG islands and the regulation of transcription. *Genes and Development, 25*, 1010–1022. 25/10/1010 [pii]. https://doi.org/10.1101/gad.2037511

Deaton, A. M., Webb, S., Kerr, A. R. W., Illingworth, R. S., Guy, J., Andrews, R., & Bird, A. (2011). Cell type–specific DNA methylation at intragenic CpG islands in the immune system. *Genome Research, 21*, 1074–1086. https://doi.org/10.1101/gr.118703.110

Dempster, E. L., Pidsley, R., Schalkwyk, L. C., Owens, S., Georgiades, A., Kane, F., … Mill, J. (2011). Disease-associated epigenetic changes in monozygotic twins discordant for schizophrenia and bipolar disorder. *Human Molecular Genetics, 20*, 4786–4796. https://doi.org/10.1093/hmg/ddr416

Docherty, S., Davis, O., Haworth, C., Plomin, R., D'Souza, U., & Mill, J. (2012). A genetic association study of DNA methylation levels in the DRD4 gene region finds associations with nearby SNPs. *Behavioral and Brain Functions, 8*, 31.

Dumais, A., Lesage, A. D., Lalovic, A., Seguin, M., Tousignant, M., Chawky, N., & Turecki, G. (2005). Is violent method of suicide a behavioral marker of lifetime aggression? *American Journal of Psychiatry, 162*, 1375–1378. https://doi.org/10.1176/appi.ajp.162.7.1375

Edgar, R. D., Jones, M. J., Meaney, M. J., Turecki, G., & Kobor, M. S. (2017). BECon: A tool for interpreting DNA methylation findings from blood in the context of brain. *bioRxiv*. https://doi.org/10.1101/111609

Edgar, R. D., Jones, M. J., Robinson, W. P., & Kobor, M. S. (2017). An empirically driven data reduction method on the human 450K methylation array to remove tissue specific non-variable CpGs. *Clinical Epigenetics, 9*, 11. https://doi.org/10.1186/s13148-017-0320-z

Esposito, E. A., Jones, M. J., Doom, J. R., MacIsaac, J. L., Gunnar, M. R., & Kobor, M. S. (2016). Differential DNA methylation in peripheral blood mononuclear cells in adolescents exposed to significant early but not later childhood adversity. *Development and Psychopathology, 28*, 1385–1399. https://doi.org/10.1017/S0954579416000055

Essex, M. J., Boyce, W. T., Hertzman, C., Lam, L. L., Armstrong, J. M., Neumann, S. M., & Kobor, M. S. (2013). Epigenetic vestiges of early developmental adversity: Childhood stress exposure and DNA methylation in adolescence. *Child Development, 84*, 58–75. https://doi.org/10.1111/j.1467-8624.2011.01641.x

Fan, G., Martinowich, K., Chin, M. H., He, F., Fouse, S. D., Hutnick, L., … Sun, Y. E. (2005). DNA methylation controls the timing of astrogliogenesis through regulation of JAK-STAT signaling. *Development, 132*, 3345–3356. https://doi.org/10.1242/dev.01912

Farre, P., Jones, M. J., Meaney, M. J., Emberly, E., Turecki, G., & Kobor, M. S. (2015). Concordant and discordant DNA methylation signatures of aging in human blood and brain. *Epigenetics & Chromatin, 8*, 19. https://doi.org/10.1186/s13072-015-0011-y

Fraga, M. F., Ballestar, E., Paz, M. F., Ropero, S., Setien, F., Ballestar, M. L., … Esteller, M. (2005). Epigenetic differences arise during the lifetime of monozygotic twins. *Proceedings of the National Academy of Sciences of the United States of America, 102*, 10604–10609. https://doi.org/10.1073/pnas.0500398102

Francis, D., Diorio, J., Liu, D., & Meaney, M. J. (1999). Nongenomic transmission across generations of maternal behavior and stress responses in the rat. *Science, 286*, 1155–1158. 7973 [pii].

Gavin, D. P., Sharma, R. P., Chase, K. A., Matrisciano, F., Dong, E., & Guidotti, A. (2012). Growth arrest and DNA-damage-inducible, Beta (GADD45b)-mediated DNA Demethylation in major psychosis. *Neuropsychopharmacology, 37*, 531–542.

Gertz, J., Varley, K. E., Reddy, T. E., Bowling, K. M., Pauli, F., Parker, S. L., … Myers, R. M. (2011). Analysis of DNA methylation in a three-generation family reveals widespread genetic influence on epigenetic regulation. *PLoS Genetics, 7*, e1002228. https://doi.org/10.1371/journal.pgen.1002228PGENETICS-D-11-00600. [pii].

Gordon, L., Joo, J. E., Powell, J. E., Ollikainen, M., Novakovic, B., Li, X., … Saffery, R. (2012). Neonatal DNA methylation profile in human twins is specified by a complex interplay between intrauterine environmental and genetic factors, subject to tissue-specific influence. *Genome Research, 22*, 1395–1406. https://doi.org/10.1101/gr.136598.111

Hackett, J. A., Sengupta, R., Zylicz, J. J., Murakami, K., Lee, C., Down, T. A., & Surani, M. A. (2013). Germline DNA demethylation dynamics and imprint erasure through 5-hydroxymethylcytosine. *Science, 339*, 448–452. https://doi.org/10.1126/science.1229277

Hannon, E., Dempster, E., Viana, J., Burrage, J., Smith, A. R., Macdonald, R., … Mill, J. (2016). An integrated genetic-epigenetic analysis of schizophrenia: Evidence for co-localization of genetic associations and differential DNA methylation. *Genome Biology, 17*, 176. https://doi.org/10.1186/s13059-016-1041-x

Hansen, K. D., Timp, W., Bravo, H. C., Sabunciyan, S., Langmead, B., McDonald, O. G., … Feinberg, A. P. (2011). Increased methylation variation in epigenetic domains across cancer types. *Nature Genetics, 43*, 768–775. https://doi.org/10.1038/ng.865

Hecker, T., Radtke, K. M., Hermenau, K., Papassotiropoulos, A., & Elbert, T. (2016). Associations among child abuse, mental health, and epigenetic modifications in the proopiomelanocortin gene (POMC): A study with children in Tanzania. *Development and Psychopathology, 28*, 1401–1412.

Heim, C., Newport, D., Jeffrey, B., Robert, M., Andrew, H., & Nemeroff, C. B. (2001). Altered pituitary-adrenal axis responses to provocative challenge tests in adult survivors of childhood abuse. *American Journal of Psychiatry, 158*, 575–581. https://doi.org/10.1176/appi.ajp.158.4.575

Hellstrom, I. C., Dhir, S. K., Diorio, J. C., & Meaney, M. J. (2012). Maternal licking regulates hippocampal glucocorticoid receptor transcription through a thyroid hormone-serotonin-NGFI-

A signalling cascade. *Philosophical Transactions of the Royal Society of London: Bioloical Sciences, 367*, 2495–2510. rstb.2012.0223 [pii]. https://doi.org/10.1098/rstb.2012.0223

Herb, B. R., Wolschin, F., Hansen, K. D., Aryee, M. J., Langmead, B., Irizarry, R., … Feinberg, A. P. (2012). Reversible switching between epigenetic states in honeybee behavioral subcastes. *Nature Neuroscience, 15*, 1371–1373. http://www.nature.com/neuro/journal/v15/n10/abs/nn.3218.html—supplementary-information.

Heyn, H., Li, N., Ferreira, H. J., Moran, S., Pisano, D. G., Gomez, A., … Esteller, M. (2012). Distinct DNA methylomes of newborns and centenarians. *Proceedings of the National Academy of Sciences of the United States of America, 109*, 10522–10527. https://doi.org/10.1073/pnas.1120658109

Holliday, R. (1989). DNA methylation and epigenetic mechanisms. *Cell Biophysics, 15*, 15–20.

Horvath, S. (2013). DNA methylation age of human tissues and cell types. *Genome Biology, 14*, R115. https://doi.org/10.1186/gb-2013-14-10-r115

Horvath, S., Zhang, Y., Langfelder, P., Kahn, R. S., Boks, M. P. M., van Eijk, K., … Ophoff, R. A. (2012). Aging effects on DNA methylation modules in human brain and blood tissue. *Genome Biology, 13*, R97.

Irizarry, R. A., Ladd-Acosta, C., Wen, B., Wu, Z., Montano, C., Onyango, P., … Feinberg, A. P. (2009). The human colon cancer methylome shows similar hypo- and hypermethylation at conserved tissue-specific CpG island shores. *Nature Genetics, 41*, 178–186. https://doi.org/10.1038/ng.298

Isagawa, K., Wang, D. F., Kobayashi, T., Itoh, T., & Maeda, R. (2011). *Development of a MEMS DC electric current sensor applicable to two-wire electrical appliance cord.* Paper presented at the Nano/Micro Engineered and Molecular Systems (NEMS), 2011 IEEE International Conference.

Jin, S.-G., Wu, X., Li, A. X., & Pfeifer, G. P. (2011). Genomic mapping of 5-hydroxymethylcytosine in the human brain. *Nucleic Acids Research, 39*, 5015–5024. https://doi.org/10.1093/nar/gkr120

Kaminsky, Z. A., Tang, T., Wang, S.-C., Ptak, C., Oh, G. H. T., Wong, A. H. C., … Petronis, A. (2009). DNA methylation profiles in monozygotic and dizygotic twins. *Nature Genetics, 41*, 240–245. http://www.nature.com/ng/journal/v41/n2/suppinfo/ng.286_S1.html

Klengel, T., Mehta, D., Anacker, C., Rex-Haffner, M., Pruessner, J. C., Pariante, C. M., … Bradley, B. (2013). Allele-specific FKBP5 DNA demethylation mediates gene-childhood trauma interactions. *Nature Neuroscience, 16*, 33–41.

Klose, R. J., & Bird, A. P. (2006). Genomic DNA methylation: The mark and its mediators. *Trends in Biochemical Sciences, 31*, 89–97.

Kriaucionis, S., & Heintz, N. (2009). The nuclear DNA base 5-Hydroxymethylcytosine is present in purkinje neurons and the brain. *Science, 324*, 929–930. https://doi.org/10.1126/science.1169786

Kumsta, R., Marzi, S. J., Viana, J., Dempster, E. L., Crawford, B., Rutter, M., … Sonuga-Barke, E. J. (2016). Severe psychosocial deprivation in early childhood is associated with increased DNA methylation across a region spanning the transcription start site of CYP2E1. *Translational Psychiatry, 6*, e830. https://doi.org/10.1038/tp.2016.95

Labonté, B., Suderman, M., Maussion, G., Navaro, L., Yerko, V., Mahar, I., … Meaney, M. J. (2012). Genome-wide epigenetic regulation by early-life trauma. *Archives of General Psychiatry, 69*, 722–731.

Lam, L. L., Emberly, E., Fraser, H. B., Neumann, S. M., Chen, E., Miller, G. E., & Kobor, M. S. (2012). Factors underlying variable DNA methylation in a human community cohort. *Proceedings of the National Academy of Sciences of the United States of America, 109(Suppl 2)*, 17253–17260. https://doi.org/10.1073/pnas.1121249109

Lappalainen, T., & Greally, J. M. (2017). Associating cellular epigenetic models with human phenotypes. *Nature Reviews Genetics, 18*, 441–451.

Levine, S. (1994). The ontogeny of the hypothalamic-pituitary-adrenal axis. The influence of maternal factors. *Annals of the New York Academy of Sciences, 746*, 275–288. https://doi.org/10.1111/j.1749-6632.1994.tb39245.x

Lienert, F., Wirbelauer, C., Som, I., Dean, A., Mohn, F., & Schubeler, D. (2011). Identification of genetic elements that autonomously determine DNA methylation states. *Nature Genetics, 43*, 1091–1097. https://doi.org/10.1038/ng.946. ng.946 [pii].

Lister, R., Mukamel, E. A., Nery, J. R., Urich, M., Puddifoot, C. A., Johnson, N. D., ... Ecker, J. R. (2013). Global epigenomic reconfiguration during mammalian brain development. *Science, 341*, 1237905. https://doi.org/10.1126/science.1237905

Liu, D., Diorio, J., Tannenbaum, B., Caldji, C., Francis, D., Freedman, A., ... Meaney, M. J. (1997). Maternal care, hippocampal glucocorticoid receptors, and hypothalamic-pituitary-adrenal responses to stress. *Science, 277*, 1659–1662.

Liu, Y., Aryee, M. J., Padyukov, L., Fallin, M. D., Hesselberg, E., Runarsson, A., ... Feinberg, A. P. (2013). Epigenome-wide association data implicate DNA methylation as an intermediary of genetic risk in rheumatoid arthritis. *Nature Biotechnology, 31*, 142–147. https://doi.org/10.1038/nbt.2487

Lu, A. T., Hannon, E., Levine, M. E., Hao, K., Crimmins, E. M., Lunnon, K., ... Horvath, S. (2016). Genetic variants near MLST8 and DHX57 affect the epigenetic age of the cerebellum. *Nature Communications, 7*, 10561.

Ma, D. K., Jang, M. H., Guo, J. U., Kitabatake, Y., Chang, M. L., Pow-Anpongkul, N., ... Song, H. (2009). Neuronal activity-induced Gadd45b promotes epigenetic DNA demethylation and adult neurogenesis. *Science, 323*(5917), 1074–1077. https://doi.org/10.1126/science.1166859

Macleod, D., Charlton, J., Mullins, J., & Bird, A. P. (1994). Sp1 sites in the mouse aprt gene promoter are required to prevent methylation of the CpG island. *Genes & Development, 8*, 2282–2292.

Marioni, R. E., Shah, S., McRae, A. F., Ritchie, S. J., Muniz-Terrera, G., Harris, S. E., ... Deary, I. J. (2015). The epigenetic clock is correlated with physical and cognitive fitness in the Lothian birth cohort 1936. *International Journal of Epidemiology, 44*, 1388–1396. https://doi.org/10.1093/ije/dyu277

Martino, D., Loke, Y. J., Gordon, L., Ollikainen, M., Cruickshank, M. N., Saffery, R., & Craig, J. M. (2013). Longitudinal, genome-scale analysis of DNA methylation in twins from birth to 18 months of age reveals rapid epigenetic change in early life and pair-specific effects of discordance. *Genome Biology, 14*, R42. https://doi.org/10.1186/gb-2013-14-5-r42

Martino, D. J., Tulic, M. K., Gordon, L., Hodder, M., Richman, T. R., Metcalfe, J., ... Saffery, R. (2011). Evidence for age-related and individual-specific changes in DNA methylation profile of mononuclear cells during early immune development in humans. *Epigenetics, 6*, 1085–1094. https://doi.org/10.4161/epi.6.9.16401

Martinowich, K., Hattori, D., Wu, H., Fouse, S., He, F., Hu, Y., ... Sun, Y. E. (2003). DNA methylation-related chromatin remodeling in activity-dependent BDNF gene regulation. *Science, 302*, 890–893. https://doi.org/10.1126/science.1090842

Maunakea, A. K., Nagarajan, R. P., Bilenky, M., Ballinger, T. J., Souza, C., Fouse, S. D., ... Costello, J. F. (2010). Conserved role of intragenic DNA methylation in regulating alternative promoters. *Nature, 466*, 253–257. http://www.nature.com/nature/journal/v466/n7303/abs/nature09165.html—supplementary-information.

Maze, I., Noh, K.-M., & Allis, C. D. (2013). Histone regulation in the CNS: Basic principles of epigenetic plasticity. *Neuropsychopharmacology, 38*, 3–22.

McGoron, L., Gleason, M. M., Smyke, A. T., Drury, S. S., Nelson, C. A., Gregas, M. C., ... Zeanah, C. H. (2012). Recovering from early deprivation: Attachment mediates effects of caregiving on psychopathology. *Journal of the American Academy of Child and Adolescent Psychiatry, 51*, 683–693. https://doi.org/10.1016/j.jaac.2012.05.004

McGowan, P. O., Sasaki, A., D'Alessio, A. C., Dymov, S., Labonte, B., Szyf, M., ... Meaney, M. J. (2009). Epigenetic regulation of the glucocorticoid receptor in human brain associates with childhood abuse. *Nature Neuroscience, 12*, 342–348.

McLaughlin, K. A., Sheridan, M. A., Winter, W., Fox, N. A., Zeanah, C. H., & Nelson, C. A. (2014). Widespread reductions in cortical thickness following severe early-life deprivation: A neurodevelopmental pathway to attention-deficit/hyperactivity disorder. *Biological Psychiatry, 76*(8), 629–638. https://doi.org/10.1016/j.biopsych.2013.08.016. S0006-3223(13)00769-5 [pii].

Meaney, M. J. (2010). Epigenetics and the biological definition of gene x environment interactions. *Child Development, 81*, 41–79. https://doi.org/10.1111/j.1467-8624.2009.01381.x. CDEV1381 [pii].

Meaney, M. J., Diorio, J., Francis, D., Weaver, S., Yau, J., Chapman, K., & Seckl, J. R. (2000). Postnatal handling increases the expression of camp-inducible transcription factors in the rat hippocampus: The effects of thyroid hormones and serotonin. *The Journal of Neuroscience, 20*, 3926–3935.

Mehta, D., Klengel, T., Conneely, K. N., Smith, A. K., Altmann, A., Pace, T. W., … Binder, E. B. (2013). Childhood maltreatment is associated with distinct genomic and epigenetic profiles in posttraumatic stress disorder. *Proceedings of the National Academy of Sciences of the United States of America, 110*, 8302–8307. https://doi.org/10.1073/pnas.1217750110

Mellén, M., Ayata, P., Dewell, S., Kriaucionis, S., & Heintz, N. (2012). MeCP2 binds to 5hmC enriched within active genes and accessible chromatin in the nervous system. *Cell, 151*(7), 1417–1430. https://doi.org/10.1016/j.cell.2012.11.022

Menard, J. L., Champagne, D. L., & Meaney, M. J. P. (2004). Variations of maternal care differentially influence 'fear' reactivity and regional patterns of cFos immunoreactivity in response to the shock-probe burying test. *Neuroscience, 129*, 297–308. https://doi.org/10.1016/j.neuroscience.2004.08.009

Mueller, B. R., & Bale, T. L. (2008). Sex-specific programming of offspring emotionality after stress early in pregnancy. *Journal of Neuroscience, 28*, 9055–9065. https://doi.org/10.1523/jneurosci.1424-08.2008

Murgatroyd, C., Patchev, A. V., Wu, Y., Micale, V., Bockmuhl, Y., Fischer, D., … Spengler, D. (2009). Dynamic DNA methylation programs persistent adverse effects of early-life stress. *Nature Neuroscience, 12*, 1559–1566. https://doi.org/10.1038/nn.2436

Nanni, V., Uher, R., & Danese, A. (2012). Childhood maltreatment predicts unfavorable course of illness and treatment outcome in depression: A meta-analysis. *American Journal of Psychiatry, 169*, 141–151.

Naumova, O. Y., Hein, S., Suderman, M., Barbot, B., Lee, M., Raefski, A., … Grigorenko, E. L. (2016). Epigenetic patterns modulate the connection between developmental dynamics of parenting and offspring psychosocial adjustment. *Child Development, 87*, 98–110.

Naumova, O. Y., Lee, M., Koposov, R., Szyf, M., Dozier, M., & Grigorenko, E. L. (2012). Differential patterns of whole-genome DNA methylation in institutionalized children and children raised by their biological parents. *Development and Psychopathology, 24*, 143–155. https://doi.org/10.1017/S0954579411000605. S0954579411000605 [pii].

Nelson, C. A., Zeanah, C. H., Fox, N. A., Marshall, P. J., Smyke, A. T., & Guthrie, D. (2007). Cognitive recovery in socially deprived young children: The Bucharest early intervention project. *Science, 318*, 1937–1940. https://doi.org/10.1126/science.1143921

Nelson, E. D., Kavalali, E. T., & Monteggia, L. M. (2008). Activity-dependent suppression of miniature neurotransmission through the regulation of DNA methylation. *The Journal of Neuroscience, 28*, 395–406. https://doi.org/10.1523/jneurosci.3796-07.2008

Non, A. L., Hollister, B. M., Humphreys, K. L., Childebayeva, A., Esteves, K., Zeanah, C. H., … Drury, S. S. (2016). DNA methylation at stress-related genes is associated with exposure to early life institutionalization. *American Journal of Physical Anthropology, 161*, 84–93. https://doi.org/10.1002/ajpa.23010

O'Connor, T. G., Rutter, M., Beckett, C., Keaveney, L., & Kreppner, J. M. (2000). The effects of global severe privation on cognitive competence: Extension and longitudinal follow-up. *Child Development, 71*, 376–390. https://doi.org/10.1111/1467-8624.00151

Papavassiliou, P., York, T. P., Gursoy, N., Hill, G., Nicely, L. V., Sundaram, U., … Jackson-Cook, C. (2009). The phenotype of persons having mosaicism for trisomy 21/Down syndrome reflects the percentage of trisomic cells present in different tissues. *American Journal of Medical Genetics, 149A*, 573–583. https://doi.org/10.1002/ajmg.a.32729

Perroud, N., Rutembesa, E., Paoloni-Giacobino, A., Mutabaruka, J., Mutesa, L., Stenz, L., … Karege, F. (2014). The Tutsi genocide and transgenerational transmission of maternal stress: Epigenetics and biology of the HPA axis. *Biological Psychiatry, 15*, 334–345.

Pidsley, R., Zotenko, E., Peters, T. J., Lawrence, M. G., Risbridger, G. P., Molloy, P., … Clark, S. J. (2016). Critical evaluation of the Illumina MethylationEPIC BeadChip microarray for whole-genome DNA methylation profiling. *Genome Biology, 17*, 208.

Provençal, N., Suderman, M. J., Guillemin, C., Massart, R., Ruggiero, A., Wang, D., … Szyf, M. (2012). The signature of maternal rearing in the methylome in rhesus macaque prefrontal cortex and T cells. *Journal of Neuroscience, 32*, 15626–15642. https://doi.org/10.1523/jneurosci.1470-12.2012

Radtke, K. M., Ruf, M., Gunter, H. M., Dohrmann, K., Schauer, M., Meyer, A., & Elbert, T. (2011). Transgenerational impact of intimate partner violence on methylation in the promoter of the glucocorticoid receptor. *Translational Psychiatry, 1*, e21. http://www.nature.com/tp/journal/v1/n7/suppinfo/tp201121s1.html

Rakyan, V. K., Down, T. A., Thorne, N. P., Flicek, P., Kulesha, E., Gräf, S., … Beck, S. (2008). An integrated resource for genome-wide identification and analysis of human tissue-specific differentially methylated regions (tDMRs). *Genome Research, 18*, 1518–1529. https://doi.org/10.1101/gr.077479.108

Razin, A., & Cedar, H. (1993). DNA methylation and embryogenesis. In *DNA methylation* (pp. 343–357). Berlin: Springer.

Razin, A., & Riggs, A. D. (1980). DNA methylation and gene function. *Science, 210*, 604–610.

Reddy, T. E., Gertz, J., Pauli, F., Kucera, K. S., Varley, K. E., Newberry, K. M., … Song, L. (2012). Effects of sequence variation on differential allelic transcription factor occupancy and gene expression. *Genome Research, 22*, 860–869.

Risch, N., Herrell, R., Lehner, T., Liang, K.-Y., Eaves, L., Hoh, J., … Merikangas, K. R. (2009). Interaction between the serotonin transporter gene (5-HTTLPR), stressful life events, and risk of depression: A meta-analysis. *Journal of the American Medical Association, 301*, 2462–2471.

Rutter, M., Kumsta, R., Schlotz, W., & Sonuga-Barke, E. (2012). Longitudinal studies using a "natural experiment" design: The case of adoptees from romanian institutions. *Journal of the American Academy of Child and Adolescent Psychiatry, 51*, 762–770. https://doi.org/10.1016/j.jaac.2012.05.011

Rutter, M., Thapar, A., & Pickles, A. (2009). Gene-environment interactions: Biologically valid pathway or artifact? *Archives of General Psychiatry, 66*, 1287–1289. https://doi.org/10.1001/archgenpsychiatry.2009.167. 66/12/1287 [pii].

Ruzov, A., Tsenkina, Y., Serio, A., Dudnakova, T., Fletcher, J., Bai, Y., … De Sousa, P. (2011). Lineage-specific distribution of high levels of genomic 5-hydroxymethylcytosine in mammalian development. *Cell Research, 21*, 1332–1342. http://www.nature.com/cr/journal/v21/n9/suppinfo/cr2011113s1.html

Sabunciyan, S., Aryee, M. J., Irizarry, R. A., Rongione, M., Webster, M. J., Kaufman, W. E., … Potash, J. B. (2012). Genome-wide DNA methylation scan in major depressive disorder. *PLoS One, 7*, e34451. https://doi.org/10.1371/journal.pone.0034451PONE-D-11-24451. [pii].

Schanberg, S. M., Evoniuk, G., & Kuhn, C. M. (1984). Tactile and nutritional aspects of maternal care: specific regulators of neuroendocrine function and cellular development. *Proceedings of the Society for Experimental Biology and Medicine, 175*, 135–146.

Schubeler, D. (2012). Molecular biology. Epigenetic islands in a genetic ocean. *Science, 338*, 756–757. https://doi.org/10.1126/science.1227243. 338/6108/756 [pii].

Shenker, N., & Flanagan, J. M. (2012). Intragenic DNA methylation: Implications of this epigenetic mechanism for cancer research. *British Journal of Cancer, 106*, 248–253.

Sheridan, M. A., Fox, N. A., Zeanah, C. H., McLaughlin, K. A., & Nelson, C. A. (2012). Variation in neural development as a result of exposure to institutionalization early in childhood. *Proceedings of the National Academy of Sciences of the United States of America, 109*, 12927–12932. https://doi.org/10.1073/pnas.1200041109

Skene, P. J., & Henikoff, S. (2013). Histone variants in pluripotency and disease. *Development, 140*, 2513–2524. https://doi.org/10.1242/dev.091439

Smith, A. K., Conneely, K. N., Kilaru, V., Mercer, K. B., Weiss, T. E., Bradley, B., ... Ressler, K. J. (2011). Differential immune system DNA methylation and cytokine regulation in post-traumatic stress disorder. *American Journal of Medical Genetics Part B: Neuropsychiatric Genetics, 156*, 700–708. https://doi.org/10.1002/ajmg.b.31212

Smith, A. K., Kilaru, V., Klengel, T., Mercer, K. B., Bradley, B., Conneely, K. N., ... Binder, E. B. (2015). DNA extracted from saliva for methylation studies of psychiatric traits: Evidence tissue specificity and relatedness to brain. *American Journal of Medical Genetics Part B: Neuropsychiatric Genetics, 168B*, 36–44. https://doi.org/10.1002/ajmg.b.32278

Sonuga-Barke, E. J. S., Kennedy, M., Kumsta, R., Knights, N., Golm, D., Rutter, M., ... Kreppner, J. (2017). Child-to-adult neurodevelopmental and mental health trajectories after early life deprivation: The young adult follow-up of the longitudinal English and Romanian adoptees study. *Lancet, 389*, 1539–1548. https://doi.org/10.1016/S0140-6736(17)30045-4

Stadler, M. B., Murr, R., Burger, L., Ivanek, R., Lienert, F., Scholer, A., ... Schubeler, D. (2011). DNA-binding factors shape the mouse methylome at distal regulatory regions. *Nature, 480*, 490–495. https://doi.org/10.1038/nature10716

Szulwach, K. E., Li, X., Li, Y., Song, C-X., Wu, H., Dai, Q., ... Jin, P. (2011). 5-hmC-mediated epigenetic dynamics during postnatal neurodevelopment and aging. *Nature Neuroscience, 14*, 1607–1616. http://www.nature.com/neuro/journal/v14/n12/abs/nn.2959.html—supplementary-information.

Szyf, M., Weaver, I. C. G., Champagne, F. A., Diorio, J., & Meaney, M. J. (2005). Maternal programming of steroid receptor expression and phenotype through DNA methylation in the rat. *Frontiers in Neuroendocrinology, 26*, 139–162.

Teh, A. L., Pan, H., Lin, X., Lim, Y., Ives, P., Chinari, P. K., ... Meaney, M. J. (2016). Comparison of methyl-capture sequencing vs. Infinium 450K methylation array for methylome analysis in clinical samples. *Epigenetics, 11*, 36–48.

Toki, S., Morinobu, S., Imanaka, A., Yamamoto, S., Yamawaki, S., & Honma, K.-I. (2007). Importance of early lighting conditions in maternal care by dam as well as anxiety and memory later in life of offspring. *European Journal of Neuroscience, 25*, 815–829. https://doi.org/10.1111/j.1460-9568.2007.05288.x

Trickett, P. K., Noll, J. G., Susman, E. J., Shenk, C. E., & Putnam, F. W. (2010). Attenuation of cortisol across development for victims of sexual abuse. *Development and Psychopathology, 22*, 165–175. https://doi.org/10.1017/S0954579409990332

Trickett, P. K., Noll, J. G., & Putnam, F. W. (2011). The impact of sexual abuse on female development: Lessons from a multigenerational, longitudinal research study. *Development and Psychopathology, 23*(02), 453–476. https://doi.org/10.1017/S0954579411000174

Turecki, G., & Meaney, M. J. (2014). Effects of the social environment and stress on glucocorticoid receptor gene methylation: A systematic review. *Biological Psychiatry, 79*, 87. https://doi.org/10.1016/j.biopsych.2014.11.022

Turner, B. M. (2001). *Chromatin and gene regulation: Mechanisms in epigenetics*. Cambridge, MA: Blackwell Science.

Turner, J. D., & Muller, C. P. (2005). Structure of the glucocorticoid receptor (NR3C1) gene 5′ untranslated region: Identification, and tissue distribution of multiple new human exon 1. *Journal of Molecular Endocrinology, 35*, 283–292. https://doi.org/10.1677/jme.1.01822

Tyrka, A. R., Price, L. H., Marsit, C., Walters, O. C., & Carpenter, L. L. (2012). Childhood adversity and epigenetic modulation of the leukocyte glucocorticoid receptor: Preliminary findings in healthy adults. *PLoS One, 7*, e30148. https://doi.org/10.1371/journal.pone.0030148PONE-D-11-16545. [pii].

Tyrka, A. R., Ridout, K. K., & Parade, S. H. (2016). Childhood adversity and epigenetic regulation of glucocorticoid signaling genes: Associations in children and adults. *Development and Psychopathology, 28*, 1319–1331.

Tyrka, A. R., Ridout, K. K., Parade, S. H., Paquette, A., Marsit, C. J., & Seifer, R. (2015). Childhood maltreatment and methylation of FK506 binding protein 5 gene (FKBP5). *Development and Psychopathology, 27*, 1637–1645.

Ursini, G., Bollati, V., Fazio, L., Porcelli, A., Iacovelli, L., Catalani, A., … Bertolino, A. (2011). Stress-related methylation of the Catechol-O-Methyltransferase Val158 allele predicts human prefrontal cognition and activity. *Journal of Neuroscience, 31*, 6692–6698. https://doi.org/10.1523/jneurosci.6631-10.2011

Varley, K. E., Gertz, J., Bowling, K. M., Parker, S. L., Reddy, T. E., Pauli-Behn, F., … Myers, R. M. (2013). Dynamic DNA methylation across diverse human cell lines and tissues. *Genome Research, 23*, 555–567. https://doi.org/10.1101/gr.147942.112

Vijayendran, M., Beach, S., Plume, J. M., Brody, G., & Philibert, R. (2012). Effects of genotype and child abuse on DNA methylation and gene expression at the serotonin transporter. *Frontiers in Psychiatry, 3*, 55. https://doi.org/10.3389/fpsyt.2012.00055

Wang, T., Pan, Q., Lin, L., Szulwach, K. E., Song, C. X., He, C., … Li, X. (2012). Genome-wide DNA hydroxymethylation changes are associated with neurodevelopmental genes in the developing human cerebellum. *Human Molecular Genetics, 21*, 5500–5510. https://doi.org/10.1093/hmg/dds394

Weaver, I. C., D'Alessio, A. C., Brown, S. E., Hellstrom, I. C., Dymov, S., Sharma, S., … Meaney, M. J. (2007). The transcription factor nerve growth factor-inducible protein a mediates epigenetic programming: Altering epigenetic marks by immediate-early genes. *Journal of Neuroscience, 27*, 1756–1768. https://doi.org/10.1523/JNEUROSCI.4164-06.2007

Weaver, I. C. G., Cervoni, N., Champagne, F. A., D'Alessio, A. C., Sharma, S., Seckl, J. R., … Meaney, M. J. (2004). Epigenetic programming by maternal behavior. *Nature Neuroscience, 7*, 847–854. http://www.nature.com/neuro/journal/v7/n8/suppinfo/nn1276_S1.html

Widom, C. S., DuMont, K., & Czaja, S. J. (2007). A prospective investigation of major depressive disorder and comorbidity in abused and neglected children grown up. *Archives of General Psychiatry, 64*, 49–56.

Wong, C. C. Y., Meaburn, E. L., Ronald, A., Price, T. S., Jeffries, A. R., Schalkwyk, L. C., … Mill, J. (2013). Methylomic analysis of monozygotic twins discordant for autism spectrum disorder and related behavioural traits. *Molecular Psychiatry, 19*, 495. https://doi.org/10.1038/mp.2013.41

Xiao, S., Xie, D., Cao, X., Yu, P., Xing, X., Chen, C. C., … Zhong, S. (2012). Comparative epigenomic annotation of regulatory DNA. *Cell, 149*, 1381–1392. https://doi.org/10.1016/j.cell.2012.04.029. S0092-8674(12)00574-0 [pii].

Yang, B.-Z., Zhang, H., Ge, W., Weder, N., Douglas-Palumberi, H., Perepletchikova, F., … Kaufman, J. (2013). Child abuse and epigenetic mechanisms of disease risk. *American Journal of Preventive Medicine, 44*, 101–107. https://doi.org/10.1016/j.amepre.2012.10.012

Yehuda, R., Daskalakis, N. P., Bierer, L. M., Bader, H. N., Klengel, T., Holsboer, F., & Binder, E. B. (2016). Holocaust exposure induced intergenerational effects on FKBP5 methylation. *Biological Psychiatry, 80*, 372–380.

Yehuda, R., Flory, J. D., Bierer, L. M., Henn-Haase, C., Lehrner, A., Desarnaud, F., … Meaney, M. J. (2014). Lower methylation of glucocorticoid receptor gene promoter 1 in peripheral blood of veterans with posttraumatic stress disorder. *Biological Psychiatry, 77*, 356. https://doi.org/10.1016/j.biopsych.2014.02.006

Yehuda, R., Flory, J. D., Bierer, L. M., Henn-Haase, C., Lehrner, A., Desarnaud, F., … Meaney, M. J. (2015). Lower methylation of glucocorticoid receptor gene promoter 1 F in peripheral blood of veterans with posttraumatic stress disorder. *Biological Psychiatry, 77*, 356–364.

Zannas, A. S., Arloth, J., Carrillo-Roa, T., Iurato, S., Roh, S., Ressler, K. J., … Mehta, D. (2015). Lifetime stress accelerates epigenetic aging in an urban, African American cohort: Relevance of glucocorticoid signaling. *Genome Biology, 16*, 266. https://doi.org/10.1186/s13059-015-0828-5

Zhang, D., Cheng, L., Badner, J. A., Chen, C., Chen, Q., Luo, W., … Liu, C. (2010). Genetic control of individual differences in gene-specific methylation in human brain. *American Journal of Human Genetics, 86*, 411–419. https://doi.org/10.1016/j.ajhg.2010.02.005. S0002-9297(10)00087-X [pii].

Zhang, T. Y., Hellstrom, I. C., Bagot, R. C., Wen, X., Diorio, J., & Meaney, M. J. (2010). Maternal care and DNA methylation of a glutamic acid decarboxylase 1 promoter in rat hippocampus. *The Journal of Neuroscience, 30*, 13130–13137. https://doi.org/10.1523/JNEUROSCI.1039-10.2010

Ziller, M. J., Gu, H., Muller, F., Donaghey, J., Tsai, L. T., Kohlbacher, O., ... Meissner, A. (2013). Charting a dynamic DNA methylation landscape of the human genome. *Nature, 500*, 477–481. https://doi.org/10.1038/nature12433

Zouk, H., Tousignant, M., Seguin, M., Lesage, A., & Turecki, G. (2006). Characterization of impulsivity in suicide completers: Clinical, behavioral and psychosocial dimensions. *Journal of Affective Disorders, 92*, 195–204.

Chapter 8
An Integrative Temporal Framework for Psychological Resilience

Kan Long and George A. Bonanno

Life can be demanding. Most people are exposed to at least one and sometimes several potentially traumatic events (PTEs) during the course of their lifetime (Breslau, 2009; Copeland, Keeler, Angold, & Costello, 2007; Norris, 1992). Importantly, however, it is now well understood that responses to adversity are characterized by significant variability. In the past decade, a growing body of research has examined these separable patterns of psychological adjustment and illustrated that human beings are, in part, defined by a capacity for resilience in the face of highly aversive events.

Researchers first became interested in resilience during the early 1970s, and the term was initially proposed to explain the process by which ecological systems absorbed "change and disturbance" (Holling, 1973, p. 14). At the same time, the concept of psychological resilience also began to emerge in the literature on early human development (Garmezy, 1972; Rutter, 1979; Werner, Bierman, & French, 1971; Werner & Smith, 1977). Although developmental psychology in this era primarily focused on psychopathology, psychological resilience served as a descriptor for children who had endured recurrent and chronic adversity, yet grew into functional, capable individuals (DiRago & Vaillant, 2007; Gralinski-Bakker, Hauser, Stott, Billings, & Allen, 2004; Sampson & Laub, 1992; Vaillant & Davis, 2000). By the early 1990s, researchers and theorists concerned with trauma exposure and psychological health in adults began to show interest in the idea of psychological resilience, which led to the advent of a different perspective on the construct (Bonanno, Papa, & O'Neill, 2001; Bonanno, Keltner, Holen, & Horowitz, 1995; Bonanno, Field, Kovacevic, & Kaltman, 2002; Ryff & Singer, 2002). Namely, research on trauma and adversity in adults has tended to focus on single, isolated events such as loss, trauma, or disaster occurring in otherwise normative environments—a trend

K. Long (✉) · G. A. Bonanno
Department of Counseling and Clinical Psychology, Teachers College, Columbia University, New York, NY, USA
e-mail: ktl2115@columbia.edu; gab38@columbia.edu

© Springer International Publishing AG, part of Springer Nature 2018

J. G. Noll, I. Shalev (eds.), *The Biology of Early Life Stress*, Child Maltreatment Solutions Network, https://doi.org/10.1007/978-3-319-72589-5_8

that diverges from the emphasis on chronic adversity and life course outcomes that is characteristic of developmental research. Thus, when researchers and theorists turned their attention towards resilience in trauma-exposed adult populations, the conceptual focus began to shift from distal psychological outcomes occurring in the extended aftermath of exposure to more proximal patterns of mental health and psychological adjustment (Bonanno et al., 2001; Bonanno, 2004, 2005; Bonanno, Westphal, & Mancini, 2011).

While the scientific evidence is most robust with regard to psychological resilience in individuals (Bonanno, Romero, & Klein, 2015), the concept has also expanded to include a wider range of social constructs and behaviors germane to families (Hawley & DeHaan, 1996; Patterson, 1988, 2002; Walsh, 1996) and communities (Norris, Stevens, Pfefferbaum, Wyche, & Pfefferbaum, 2008; Sonn & Fisher, 1998). For instance, psychological resilience in family systems has involved family communication patterns (McCubbin & McCubbin, 1988), family problem solving and flexibility (Walsh, 1996), and family identity (Patterson, 2002). Concurrently, prior work on resilience in communities integrates sense of community (Sonn & Fisher, 1998), social capital (Kawachi, 1999), and collective efficacy (Sampson, Raudenbush, & Earls, 1997).

The increasing prominence of psychological resilience across divergent literatures in conjunction with a proliferation of research and theory has led to a significantly broadened definition of the term (Bonanno et al., 2015; Luthar, Cicchetti, & Becker, 2000). The current state of affairs is such that resilience has become associated with a multitude of different meanings in a variety of contexts. For example, psychological resilience has been defined as the interactive process by which positive adaptation is cultivated and maintained (Egeland, Carlson, & Sroufe, 1993; Norris et al., 2008), a post-PTE outcome characterized by healthy functioning and adjustment (e.g., Bonanno, 2004; Masten, 2007; Norris, Tracy, & Galea, 2009; Rutter, 2002), a personality trait (e.g., a "resilient" type; Smith et al., 2008), or a cluster of capacities, characteristics, and resources (Aldrich, 2012; Norris et al., 2008). Additional conceptual diversity arises from the application of the term resilience in reference to both acute and chronic life stressors (Bonanno & Diminich, 2013) as well as a variety of populations that includes children (Masten, 2001), adults (Bonanno, 2004), families (Walsh, 2006, 2013), and neighborhoods or communities (Norris et al., 2008).

However, when "resilience" is used in isolation to describe a single construct, the collection of varying and overlapping meanings lacks sufficient conceptual and scientific precision to drive continued inquiry. In the interest of integrating the disparate literature on psychological resilience, we propose that the concept of resilience is best realized as a broad, umbrella phenomenon that encompasses a number of temporally related elements (Bonanno, 2004, 2005; Bonanno & Diminich, 2013; Carver, 1998; Cutter et al., 2008; Masten & Narayan, 2012; Norris et al., 2008). In the following sections, we review a recent, novel framework that endeavors to organize and advance research and theory on psychological resilience.

8.1 An Integrative Temporal Framework

Bonanno et al. (2015) proposed an integrative temporal framework that sought common threads among the vast literature on resilience in individuals, families, and communities. The authors argued that the study of resilience across diverse fields should necessarily reference four constituent temporal elements (Fig. 8.1). These four elements include: (a) baseline or pre-adversity adjustment that serves as the anchoring reference point, (b) the actual aversive circumstances, (c) post-adversity resilient outcomes referenced to both the aversive circumstances and baseline adjustment, and (d) predictors of resilient outcomes measured prior to, during, and after the aversive circumstances. In the context of this framework, psychological resilience is conceptualized as a process that unfolds over time (Bonanno, 2012).

8.1.1 Aversive Circumstances

The first temporal element to define is the aversive circumstances themselves. Despite the temporal precedence of baseline adjustment, it is essential to begin by asking "resilience to what?" (Bonanno et al., 2015, p. 141). In other words,

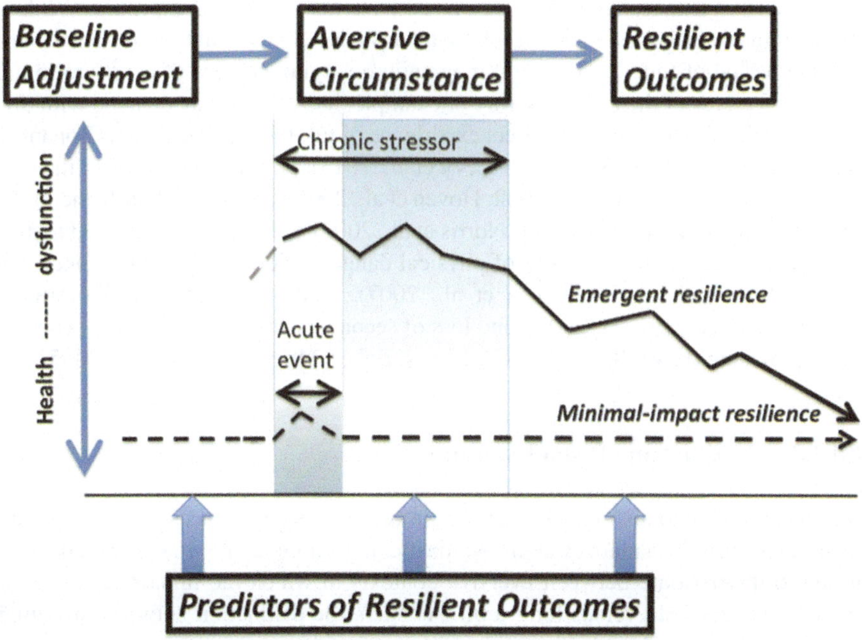

Fig. 8.1 The temporal elements of psychological resilience. From Bonanno, G. A., Romero, S. A., & Klein, S. I. (2015). The temporal elements of psychological resilience: An integrative framework for the study of individuals, families, and communities. *Psychological Inquiry 26*(2), 139–169

psychological resilience must be referenced to an actual real-world event or series of events (Bonanno, 2004, 2012; Luthar et al., 2000), and aversive circumstances may be distinguished on the basis of three primary features.

8.1.1.1 Acute and Chronic Events

A key distinction can be made between acute and chronic adversity. Generally speaking, acute and chronic events differ with regard to the intensity and duration of impact (Bonanno, 2004; Fergus & Zimmerman, 2004). Acute adversity involves an event that is relatively isolated, demands and/or results in the loss of resources, and exerts its primary impact over a transient period, typically less than 1 month. For example, acute events may include a natural disaster, serious transportation accident, physical assault, terrorist attack, explosion, or fire. In contrast, chronic adversity refers to an event or series of events that exert a recurrent and cumulative impact on resources and adaptation over the course of many months or years. Chronic events may consist of emotional or physical neglect, prolonged physical or sexual abuse, civil war, and political violence.

8.1.1.2 Level of Exposure

Aversive circumstances may also be parsed in terms of level of exposure. While a group of individuals can experience the same instance of potential trauma over a comparable period of time, each person may endure varying degrees of exposure to the aversive features of the event. By way of example, individuals may contend with differing levels of exposure to the direct experience of life-threatening events (Bonanno, Rennicke, & Dekel, 2005; Galatzer-Levy et al., 2013), physical proximity to the epicenter of an event (Galea et al., 2002; Hoven et al., 2005), and loss of family members or friends as the result of an event (Norris et al., 2002). Other common characteristics of exposure include the presence of physical dangers (Norris et al., 2002; Okumura et al., 1998) and injuries (Galea et al., 2007), media consumption (Vasterman, Yzermans, & Dirkzwager, 2005), and loss of secondary resources related to property or employment (Hobfoll, 1989, 2002; Norris, Baker, Murphy, & Kaniasty, 2005).

8.1.1.3 Proximal and Distal Exposure

It is also possible to distinguish aversive circumstances on the basis of proximal and distal exposure. Bonanno, Brewin, Kaniasty, and La Greca (2010) proposed these terms to differentiate between aversive contexts in which the impact of potential trauma is immediate versus long-term. As such, the distinction between proximal and distal exposure largely serves to denote *when* the impact of a highly aversive event is most prominent. Proximal exposure refers to the events and consequences that occur during the approximate period of adversity, such as imminent physical danger or the death and serious injury of others as the event unfolds. By contrast, distal exposure refers to the events and consequences that emerge in the aftermath of adversity—specifically, the lingering consequences that may take the form of prolonged injuries, displacement or relocation, and repeated repercussive events that interfere with daily functioning.

8.1.2 Baseline Adjustment

The second temporal element to establish is baseline or pre-adversity adjustment. Baseline adjustment refers to the pre-existing or baseline functioning of individuals, families, or communities prior to the onset of aversive circumstances. Almost all theories of resilience reference baseline adjustment either explicitly, in their measurements, or implicitly in their conceptual approach. In principle, resilience implies some previous level of psychological adjustment from which the response to adversity is referenced.

Prospective and longitudinal research on resilience in the face of highly aversive events has provided compelling evidence for the importance of baseline measures, by demonstrating that such inclusive designs reduce issues of sampling and memory bias (Galatzer-Levy, Huang, & Bonanno, 2017), thereby allowing for more reliable and comprehensive conclusions to be drawn. We note, however, that although it is preferable to obtain an index of psychological adjustment at baseline, the task poses notable challenges, and many situations arise in which pre-event assessments are either not feasible or available. In cases in which the acquisition of such measures is not possible, it becomes all the more critical that researchers subject measures of post-event resilient outcomes to careful scrutiny.

8.1.3 Resilient Outcomes

The third temporal element to delineate consists of post-adversity resilient outcomes. Resilient outcomes refer to the functioning of individuals, families, or communities following aversive circumstances in the aftermath of exposure (i.e., post-adversity psychological adjustment).

To date, the two most common approaches to studying highly aversive and potentially traumatic life events have employed either a binary focus on psychopathology or average-level measures of psychological adjustment. The first of these approaches has been referred to as the *diagnostic approach* and centers on the assumption that diagnostic categories reflecting the presence and absence of psychopathology (i.e., extreme responses) fully capture possible responses to adversity. As such, a diagnosis of Posttraumatic Stress Disorder (PTSD), Major Depressive Disorder (MDD), or Complicated Grief (CG) is thought to be indicative of a dysfunctional or abnormal response while the absence of psychopathology is interpreted as a normal or resilient response (e.g., Krystal & Neumeister, 2009; Rutter, 1985; Sarapas et al., 2011; Yehuda & Flory, 2007).

Research on psychopathology conducted under the auspices of the diagnostic approach has been instrumental in chronicling the adverse consequences and public health costs of exposure to potential trauma. Despite recognition of the potentially harmful effects of trauma exposure in the early twentieth century, controversy abounded regarding the presentation, prevalence, and existence of trauma-related disorders (Lamprecht & Sack, 2002). Further, the stigmatization of psychological issues experienced in the wake of potential trauma contributed to a scarcity of available treatments (Shepard, 2001). When PTSD was formally recognized as a diagnostic category in 1980, this critical turning point resulted in a significant expansion of research and treatment (Foa & Kozak, 1986; Foa, Rothbaum, Riggs, & Murdock, 1991; McNally, 2003). Recently, similar advances have taken place in the field of bereavement following the proposal of diagnostic criteria for CG (Boelen, de Keijser, van den Hout, & van den Bout, 2007; Bonanno et al., 2007; Horowitz et al., 1997; Prigerson et al., 2009; Shear, Frank, Houck, & Reynolds, 2005).

While these advances provided a foundation for our understanding of how individuals respond to adversity, the diagnostic approach is limited in several ways. The exclusive reliance on diagnostic categories results in ambiguity regarding the prevalence or course of extreme responses. In particular, one crucial problem posed by the diagnostic approach is the considerable variability in the prevalence rates of psychopathology across studies, which is most likely derived from a lack of diagnostic precision and selection or response biases (Bonanno et al., 2010; Johnson & Thompson, 2008). A historical examination of trauma research indicates significant variability in the manifestation of PTSD symptoms (Jones, 2006; Jones & Wessely, 2005; Jones et al., 2003; Sundin, Fear, Iversen, Rona, & Wessely, 2010), and clear boundaries for the diagnostic category have remained elusive (McNally, 2012). Indeed, the continued expansion of diagnostic criteria for PTSD geared towards accommodating a greater emphasis on the subjective experience of trauma has led to a form of "bracket creep" that may reduce the validity of the diagnosis (McNally, 2003, 2012). A particularly compelling illustration can be found in the current DSM-5 criteria for PTSD that allows for 636,120 separate symptom combinations qualifying for the same diagnosis (Galatzer-Levy & Bryant, 2013).

Another issue is that the binary conceptualization of psychological outcomes offers scant information regarding the distribution of responses to adversity. When all individuals who do not develop psychopathology following exposure are placed into a single category of non-psychopathology, any existing variation becomes obscured by the conflation of resilient outcomes with other non-pathological responses (Bonanno et al., 2011). In this way, the psychopathology approach presumes that the course of post-adversity outcomes follows a single *homogenous* pattern over time (Duncan, Duncan, & Strycker, 2006; Muthén, 2004). However, more recent work examining the range of responses to aversive events has consistently demonstrated *heterogeneity* in outcomes and significant variation among individuals (Bonanno, 2004; Bonanno et al., 2011; Galatzer-Levy & Bonanno, 2013).

The second approach has been termed the *average-level approach* and makes use of average-level data on psychological adjustment in order to examine differences between the mean response in a group of exposed individuals and a comparison group (e.g., non-exposed individuals or another patient population). The impact of the aversive event itself is of greatest interest in the context of the average-level approach as opposed to that of potential individual differences. Typically, the pattern of PTSD symptoms averaged at the group level takes the form of an initial elevation in the weeks immediately following exposure, which is then succeeded by a gradual decline over the course of several years and an eventual return to the assumed baseline (Breslau, 2001). The use of average-level scores has been frequently applied in studies examining predictors of PTSD or CG, and the approach has facilitated meta-analytic research involving the synthesis of information across several data sets (Currier, Neimeyer, & Berman, 2008; Norris et al., 2002).

Yet, the assumption inherent to the average-level approach is that the statistical mean reflects the normal or modal response to adversity, which represents a significant limitation. While the approach provides a description of the outcome distribution and allows for an identification of longitudinal trends, the use of average-level data may mask other interesting effects (Bloembergen & Zewail, 1984; Siegler, 1987). This issue is of particular concern to the study of psychological adjustment in the presence of adversity as the data are often non-normal, and thus the use of averages can be misleading.

It is ultimately essential to collect repeated and longitudinal measurements in order to accurately assess resilient outcomes and to model the marked variability in responses to adversity over time (Bonanno, 2012). However, the average-level approach fails to capture the heterogeneity of longitudinal distributions and is unable to identify resilient trajectories or other patterns in the data that are not encapsulated by the single, average pattern of change (Mancini, Bonanno, & Clark, 2011; Galatzer-Levy & Bonanno, 2012, 2014).

8.1.3.1 The Trajectory Approach

A burgeoning line of research has employed latent growth modeling methods (e.g., latent growth mixture modeling, latent class growth analysis) that address the limitations inherent to the diagnostic and average-level approaches by identifying trajectories of psychological adjustment. In this way, the trajectory approach more successfully models the heterogeneity in responses to highly aversive events over time. Across numerous studies, four prototypical trajectories of psychological adjustment have consistently emerged: chronic dysfunction, recovery, delayed reactions, and resilience (e.g., Bonanno, 2004, 2005; Bonanno et al., 2011). A comparison across different age groups and types of aversive circumstances has revealed two distinct resilient trajectories—*emergent resilience* and *minimal-impact resilience* (Bonanno & Diminich, 2013). These two forms of resilience are associated with distinct aversive circumstances: emergent resilience has been observed in the context of chronic adversity and minimal-impact resilience has been identified following acute adversity. Additionally, prior work has tended to link emergent resilience with developmental populations and minimal-impact resilience with adult populations. It should be noted, however, that the relationship between type of resilience and age is most likely tied to the differing interests of developmental and adult researchers, with the former emphasizing chronic aversive events and the latter focusing on acute aversive events.

8.1.3.2 Emergent Resilience

The trajectory of emergent resilience is characterized by a capacity for weathering caustic life circumstances as evidenced by the ability to reach normal developmental milestones and attain psychological health in the aftermath of chronic adversity. Given that chronic adversity can exert enduring effects on a broad spectrum of psychological and physiological functions (de Kloet, Derijk, & Meijer, 2011; Lupien, McEwen, Gunnar, & Heim, 2009; Offidani & Ruini, 2012), emergent resilience often becomes most apparent once the aversive circumstances have subsided. For instance, a child may experience ongoing difficulties within a chronically abusive family system. Yet, this same child could go on to exhibit a pattern of emergent resilience if he or she were to eventually achieve normal developmental milestones as well as exhibit healthy psychological adjustment and other age-appropriate competencies (Elder, 1998; Luthar et al., 2000; Masten & Coatsworth, 1998; Waters & Sroufe, 1983).

Much of the prior work on emergent resilience has involved the examination of chronic exposure to poverty or abuse (Garmezy, 1993; Luthar, 1999; Werner, 1993) and civil war, among other aversive circumstances (Betancourt & Khan, 2008; Betancourt, McBain, Newnham, & Brennan, 2013) in developmental populations. One classic study of emergent resilience investigated life course outcomes in a multiracial cohort of children exposed to perinatal stress, chronic poverty, chronic familial discord, and parental psychopathology (Werner, 1993, 1995; Werner & Smith, 1977, 1992). Children entered the study as newborns and were assessed over an extended period of 32 years. By late adolescence, children that demonstrated emergent resilience were observed to be competent, caring, and motivated as well as successful in several domains including academic endeavors and social functioning (Werner, 1993). Upon reaching adulthood, the majority of the resilient individuals continued to evidence adaptation and healthy psychological adjustment as indicated by scholastic and professional achievements that surpassed their high-risk peers and were comparable to the accomplishments of low-risk peers who had developed in more stable environments (Werner, 1993).

Another compelling example of emergent resilience can be found in a more recent study that examined the trajectories of internalizing symptoms and behavioral problems in Sierra Leonean youth exposed to the decade-long civil war (Betancourt et al., 2013). In this sample of war-exposed children and adolescents that included a large proportion of former child soldiers, the pattern most commonly observed was emblematic of emergent resilience and consisted of moderately elevated to highly elevated symptoms that gradually approached normal levels only after several years had passed.

It is relevant to note that even though prior work on emergent resilience is most prominent in the developmental psychology literature, this type of resilience is not limited solely to adverse experiences in childhood. Although the majority of research in adults concerns itself with acute PTEs, previous studies from the adult literature that investigated psychological adaption and functioning in the context of chronic adversity have similarly reported emergent resilient outcomes. One study, in particular, examined the impact of chronic exposure to the *Second Intifada* in a large sample of Palestinian adults from the Gaza and West Bank regions (Hobfoll et al., 2011). The most common response to extreme war violence and mass casualty involved a trajectory of moderately elevated symptoms of PTSD and depression followed by gradual improvement indicative of emergent resilience.

8.1.3.3 Minimal-Impact Resilience

The trajectory of minimal-impact resilience is characterized by a pattern of low-level, transient psychological symptoms or distress that remains stable before and after the aversive event (Bonanno, 2004, 2005; Bonanno et al., 2011). Under conditions of acute adversity, the relatively discrete and isolated nature of events typically precipitates transient disruptions in normal functioning followed by a fairly rapid return to baseline adjustment (e.g., Bisconti, Bergeman, & Boker, 2004; Bonanno, 2004). Thus, minimal-impact resilience tends to become apparent shortly after an acute aversive event occurs.

The corpus of evidence for minimal-impact resilience has arisen predominantly from research in adult populations (Bonanno & Diminich, 2013; Bonanno et al., 2015), and across many different types of PTEs, minimal-impact resilience is the most commonly observed outcome. For instance, the minimal-impact resilience trajectory was identified in the context of exposure to a large-scale terrorist attack (Bonanno et al., 2005), disease epidemic (Bonanno et al., 2008), natural disaster (La Greca et al., 2013; Norris et al., 2009; Pietrzak, Van Ness, Fried, Galea, & Norris, 2013; Tang, 2007), mass shooting (Mancini, Littleton, & Grills, 2016; Orcutt, Bonanno, Hannan, & Miron, 2014), police service (Galatzer-Levy, Madan, Neylan, Henn-Haase, & Marmar, 2011), and military deployment (Andersen, Karstoft, Bertelsen, & Madsen, 2014; Berntsen et al., 2012; Bonanno et al., 2012; Porter et al., 2017). The same pattern of stable, low-level psychological symptoms was found following bereavement (Bonanno, Field, et al., 2002; Maccallum, Galatzer-Levy, & Bonanno, 2015), divorce (Malgaroli, Galatzer-Levy, & Bonanno, 2017; Mancini et al., 2011), and job loss (Mancini et al., 2011). In addition, minimal-impact resilience was also observed in the wake of highly aversive medical events such as traumatic injury (Bombardier, Hoekstra, Dikmen, & Fann, 2016; Bonanno, Mancini, et al., 2012; deRoon-Cassini, Mancini, Bonanno, & Rusch, 2010), cancer diagnosis (Burton, Galatzer-Levy, & Bonanno, 2015; Deshields, Tibbs, Fan, & Taylor, 2006; Helgeson, Snyder, & Seltman, 2004; Lam et al., 2010), heart attack (Galatzer-Levy & Bonanno, 2014), and chronic pain (Zhu, Galatzer-Levy, & Bonanno, 2014).

As a complement to the preponderance of research on minimal-impact resilience in adult populations, recent developmental work has also identified this type of resilience in children and adolescents exposed to acute aversive events (Hong et al., 2014; La Greca et al., 2013; Le Brocque, Hendrikz, & Kenardy, 2010). In a large sample of children hospitalized for both life-threatening and benign injuries, the modal response was a stable trajectory of low-level posttraumatic stress symptoms that mirrored patterns of minimal-impact resilience observed in adults who had experienced traumatic injury (e.g., deRoon-Cassini et al., 2010). A similar study examined PTSD symptoms in a diverse group of children from New Orleans who were exposed to Hurricane Katrina (Self-Brown, Lai, Thompson, McGill, & Kelley, 2013). The children were assessed at 3, 13, 19, and 25 months post-Katrina and across the sample, and the majority of the disaster-exposed youth exhibited the minimal-impact resilience trajectory.

8.1.4 Predictors of Resilient Outcomes

The fourth and final temporal element to elucidate includes predictors of resilient outcomes. While myriad factors are touted as resilience promoting and cited as descriptors or measures of the construct, the association between these factors and resilient outcomes often derives from an assumption made on the basis of theory or clinical observation as opposed to empirical study. In the literature on families and communities, the relationship between factors and resilient outcomes has yet to be directly tested and, thus, a corresponding gap in the evidence exists. As a point of contrast, this issue is much less prominent in the literature on individual resilience by virtue of a robust body of studies that has consistently and even prospectively linked predictors with resilient outcomes.

Previous reviews have catalogued the scientific evidence for predictors of individual resilience in children (Cicchetti & Rogosch, 2012; Fergus & Zimmerman, 2004; Luthar, 2003; Ong, Bergeman, & Boker, 2009; Werner, 1995) and adults (Bonanno, 2004; Bonanno et al., 2011; Reich, Zautra, & Hall, 2010), as well as provided a synthesis of the literature across age groups (Bonanno & Diminich, 2013; Masten & Narayan, 2012). Together, these systematic reviews have identified key predictors empirically linked to resilient outcomes and highlighted two essential points. The first point concerns the primacy of single predictors. While a diverse set of variables is consistently and reliably associated with resilience, no single predictor exerts a dominant influence. Rather, each unique factor appears to exert relatively small effects by independently explaining a modest amount of the overall variance in resilient outcomes (e.g., Bonanno, Galea, Bucciarelli, & Vlahov, 2007; Werner, 1985). The second point is related to the shifting role of predictors over time. The matrix of risk and resilience factors is not static, but rather fluid and likely to change (Bonanno et al., 2010). Some predictors of resilient outcomes will remain reasonably stable with the passage of time, such as those related to personality traits, while others will fluctuate in concert with changing life circumstances and the availability of personal or situational resources (Hobfoll, 1989, 2002).

8.1.5 Predictors of Emergent Resilience

8.1.5.1 Caregiver–Child Relationships

One pertinent category of predictors is related to characteristics of the caregiver–child relationship. Aspects of the parent–child relationship that predict emergent resilient outcomes include a stable living situation, a consistent and constructive parental disciplinary style, and a nurturing parent–child dynamic (Conger & Conger, 1992, 2002; DuMont, Widom, & Czaja, 2007; Masten et al., 1999; Werner, 1993; Wyman et al., 1992). Because chronic adversity often takes a toll on the relationship between parents and children, supportive relationships with substitute caregivers (e.g., a grandparent, older sibling, or adult outside of the immediate family) have also been implicated in emergent resilience (Conger & Conger, 2002; Flores, Cicchetti, & Rogosch, 2005; Rutter, 1979; Werner, 1995).

8.1.5.2 Personal Qualities, Cognitive Skills, and Emotion

Several individual characteristics have been tied to emergent resilient outcomes. Personal qualities including self-esteem and positive self-image have been associated with resilience in the context of childhood adversity (Cicchetti & Rogosch, 1997; DuMont & Provost, 1999; Flores et al., 2005; Werner, 1995; Wyman et al., 1992). In the cognitive domain, higher intelligence (Masten et al., 1999) as well as better-developed readings skills (Werner, 1993) and problem-solving abilities (DuMont & Provost, 1999; Werner, 1995) have also characterized individuals who demonstrated emergent resilience. In addition, patterns of emotion have similarly been associated with psychological adjustment and functioning in the presence of chronic adversity (Werner & Smith, 1982; Cicchetti & Rogosch, 2009; Cicchetti, Rogosch, Lynch, & Holt, 1993).

8.1.5.3 Flexibility

Another class of predictors relevant to emergent resilience is flexibility in cognitive processes and emotion regulation (Cicchetti & Rogosch, 1997; Flores et al., 2005). In a longitudinal study of Palestinian children exposed to potential trauma during and after the *First Intifada* period, results revealed that cognitive flexibility was unrelated to psychological adjustment when traumatic exposure was at its highest level and instead served as a long-term buffer (Qouta, El-Sarraj, & Punamäki, 2001). Among children who experienced the highest levels of exposure, greater cognitive flexibility predicted healthier psychological adjustment 3 years later. The construct of flexibility will be discussed further in the section on predictors of minimal-impact resilience.

8.1.5.4 Genes

Research on gene-by-environment interactions in the context of chronic adversity has continued to expand in recent years (Nugent et al., 2011), and thus far, several gene polymorphisms have been linked to emergent resilient outcomes. More specifically, previous research has demonstrated that variation in the serotonin transporter gene (5-HTTLPR), oxytocin (OXTR) and dopamine (DRD4-521C/T) receptor genes, and the corticotropin-releasing hormone receptor gene (CRHR1) moderated the effects of childhood maltreatment in individuals who exhibited patterns of emergent resilience (Cicchetti & Rogosch, 2012).

8.1.6 Predictors of Minimal-Impact Resilience

8.1.6.1 Demographics

A host of demographic variables have been examined in previous investigations with age, gender, and race/ethnicity most frequently referenced as predictors of minimal-impact resilience.

In terms of age, relevant predictive effects exist at both early and late stages of life. Younger children were less likely to exhibit a minimal-impact resilience trajectory than older children when contending with a traumatic injury (Le Brocque et al., 2010) and experienced greater psychology difficulty than adults following exposure to a disaster (Norris et al., 2002). Older adults, in turn, demonstrated higher initial levels of distress in the presence of disasters; however, they ultimately evinced fewer long-term psychological difficulties than younger adults (Huerta & Horton, 1978; Kato, Asukai, Miyake, Minakawa, & Nishiyama, 1996; Knight, Gatz, Heller, & Bengtson, 2000) and maintained a higher probability of displaying the minimal-impact resilience trajectory upon exposure to terrorist attack and spousal loss (Bonanno, Galea, et al., 2007; Mancini et al., 2011). For its part as a predictor of minimal-impact resilience, gender appears to exert a small but reliable effect in both developmental and adult populations (Ahern, Galea, Resnick, & Vlahov, 2004; Bonanno et al., 2008; Bonanno, Galea, et al., 2007; Carr et al., 1997a, b; Hoven et al., 2005; Galea, Tracy, Norris, & Coffey, 2008; Vernberg, La Greca, Silverman, & Prinstein, 1996; Weems et al., 2010). By contrast, evidence for the predictive utility of race and ethnicity remains limited as a result of issues arising from a lack of data, racially or ethnically homogenous samples, or the presence of other confounding variables.

8.1.6.2 Social and Economic Resources

Numerous studies point to the existence of a relationship between social resources and post-PTE psychological adjustment (Brewin, Andrews, & Valentine, 2000; Kaniansty & Norris, 2009; LaGreca, Silverman, Vernberg, & Prinstein, 1996). In this regard, prior work has reported that the availability of social support and the perceived quality of this support were uniquely associated with trajectories of minimal-impact resilience following disasters (Bonanno, Galea, et al., 2007; Bonanno et al., 2008). Interestingly, prospective bereavement research found that instrumental support from family and friends (e.g., assistance with domestic or familial responsibilities) predicted minimal-impact resilient outcomes, whereas social support appeared to be less essential in buffering against the experience of loss (Bonanno et al., 2002).

While prior work supports an association between the availability of economic resources and better psychological adjustment following exposure to PTEs, this relationship has not been found in relation to trajectories of resilience (Bonanno et al., 2005; Bonanno, Galea, et al., 2007). However, the loss of resources can often be a stressor or consequence that occurs after a PTE as part of distal exposure. Previous studies have demonstrated that individuals who incurred a loss of income following the onset of aversive circumstances were less likely to exhibit the minimal-impact resilience trajectory (Bonanno, Galea, et al., 2007; Mancini et al., 2011).

8.1.6.3 Personality

While both cross-sectional and prospective studies have tested personality predictors of minimal-impact resilience, the most compelling evidence comes from prior prospective work as the assessment of personality prior to the onset of adversity addresses potential issues related to directionality (Bonanno & Mancini, 2008) and the malleability of personality depending on situational or environmental factors (McCrae et al., 2000). When measured prior to PTE exposure, low negative affectivity (Weems et al., 2007), high trait self-enhancement (Gupta & Bonanno, 2010), and a less ruminative response style (Nolen-Hoeksema & Morrow, 1991) predicted better post-PTE psychological adjustment. Similar findings were observed in relation to pre-event perceived control (Ullman & Newcomb, 1999) and trait resilience (Ong, Fuller-Rowell, & Bonanno, 2010. Several studies have also directly linked personality with the minimal-impact resilience trajectory. Quale and Schanke (2010) assessed trait coping self-efficacy, trait positive affectivity, and trait negative affectivity shortly after a traumatic injury occurred, and though the study was not truly prospective, each trait was associated with the minimal-impact resilience trajectory. Further, in a prospective study of responses to heart attack, levels of pre-event optimism obtained several years prior to the onset of a first heart attack predicted a trajectory of consistently low depression symptoms indicative of minimal-impact resilience (Galatzer-Levy & Bonanno, 2014).

8.1.6.4 Exposure

A higher degree of proximal exposure to stressors and consequences arising during the period in which a PTE occurs has been associated with increased posttraumatic stress in children (LaGreca et al., 1996) and adults (Bonanno et al., 2005; Nolen-Hoeksema & Morrow, 1991) as well as reduced prevalence rates of the minimal-impact resilience trajectory across both age groups (Bonanno et al., 2005, Bonanno, Galea, Bucciarelli, & Vlahov, 2006; Le Brocque et al., 2010). That said, the impact of exposure on rates of resilience is relatively small. For example, prospective studies of PTSD symptom trajectories in soldiers deployed for combat have consistently reported prevalence rates of minimal-impact resilience in upwards of 80% of their samples (Berntsen et al., 2012; Bonanno, Mancini, et al., 2012). A comparison of PTSD symptom trajectories between soldiers with and without significant combat exposure demonstrated that despite a modest reduction in minimal-impact resilience outcomes for those with significant combat exposure, rates of resilience remained over 80% in the exposed group (Donoho, Bonanno, Porter, Kearney, & Powell, 2017).

8.1.6.5 Past and Present Stress

A number of studies have illustrated that prior exposure to potential trauma and the presence of current life stress confers greater risk for PTSD (Brewin et al., 2000) and reduces the odds of minimal-impact resilient outcomes following PTEs (Bonanno, Galea, et al., 2007). However, the evidence is equivocal given that much of the prior work has employed retrospective measures. Although prospective data is relatively rare, Breslau, Peterson, and Schultz (2008) found that prior exposure to PTEs did not necessarily increase risk; instead, only PTEs that precipitated the development of PTSD predicted psychological adjustment upon subsequent exposure. While it seems plausible that the converse could similarly be inferred, it remains unclear whether a previous display of minimal-impact resilience following exposure to PTEs would then predict subsequent resilience.

8.1.6.6 Positive Emotion

The salutary effects of positive emotions extend across multiple contexts (Lyubomirsky, King, & Diener, 2005; Seligman & Csikszentmihalyi, 2000), and these benefits often manifest themselves most prominently in the presence of adversity (Bonanno, 2004, 2005; Moskowitz, Folkman, & Acree, 2003; Ong, Bergeman, & Chow, 2010). One prospective bereavement study reported that positive emotions mediated the relationship between spousal loss and alterations in diurnal cortisol response (Ong, Fuller-Rowell, Bonanno, & Almeida, 2011). Two separate prospective studies of 9/11 have likewise illustrated the link between positive emotion and psychological adaptation. In the first study, college students who expressed genuine smiles during a monologue about their life after the terrorist attacks following a sadness induction evinced better psychological adjustment 2 years later. In the second investigation, self-reported positive emotions mediated the relationships between pre-event ego resilience and post-event depression (Fredrickson, Tugade, Waugh, & Larkin, 2003). Recent work on trait emotion has complemented these findings by establishing that trait positive emotion functions as a prospective buffer of post-event distress with the protective effect becoming increasingly pronounced at the highest levels of exposure (Long & Bonanno, 2017).

8.1.6.7 Appraisal and Coping

Any highly aversive event may be appraised in many ways, and the nature of the interpretation can predict minimal-impact resilient outcomes (Lazarus & Folkman, 1984). The appraisal of a PTE as threatening or harmful (i.e., a threat appraisal) or as an opportunity for growth or mastery (i.e., a challenge appraisal; Ferguson, Matthews, & Cox, 1999) influences the ensuing psychological responses. Longitudinal studies of spinal cord injury found that patients who made threat appraisals experienced higher anxiety over time (Kennedy, Lude, Efström, & Smithson, 2011). Yet, patients who interpreted their spinal cord injury as a challenge to be met rather than exclusively as a threat experienced lower levels of depression. Consistent with this pattern, spinal cord injury patients who exhibited the minimal-impact resilience trajectory tended to form challenge appraisals as opposed to threat appraisals (Bonanno, Kennedy, Galatzer-Levy, Lude, & Elfström, 2012). A related factor that has been associated with long-term outcomes following PTEs is coping strategy (e.g., Nezu & Carnevale, 1987; Buckelew et al., 1990; Frank et al., 1987; Elfström, Kennedy, Lude, & Taylor, 2007; Kennedy et al., 2000). For example, resilient spinal cord patients were characterized by a proclivity towards more adaptive coping strategies involving acceptance or a "fighting spirit" rather than those related to social reliance or behavioral disengagement (Bonanno, Kennedy, et al., 2012).

8.1.6.8 Flexibility

The final category of predictors encompasses flexibility in self-regulation (Bonanno, 2005; Cheng, 2001; Kashdan & Rottenberg, 2010). This type of flexibility is of particular importance given that the characteristics and features of highly aversive events vary significantly as do the behaviors and strategies that may be most useful in these circumstances. Accordingly, regulatory flexibility refers to one's ability to adequately assess situational demands, to employ many different behaviors or strategies, and to make adjustments as the optimal strategies for a given situation change over time (Bonanno & Burton, 2013).

Coping flexibility has routinely emerged as factor that influences minimal-impact resilient outcomes. Though coping strategies are frequently labeled as either adaptive or maladaptive in the literature, the success of coping efforts primarily stems from whether or not the selected strategy is the best fit for the characteristics and demands of a situation (Aspinwall & Taylor, 1997; Block, 1993; Lazarus & Folkman, 1984). Bonanno et al. (2011) examined psychological responses to terrorist violence in a sample of Israeli college students and found that low coping flexibility was associated with higher posttraumatic stress at elevated levels of exposure, whereas high coping flexibility corresponded to relatively minimal changes in posttraumatic stress across levels of exposure (Bonanno et al., 2011). In a comparable study of PTEs in American college students, individuals exhibiting the minimal-impact resilience trajectory were more likely to use optimistic coping strategies geared towards maintaining normal goals and plans rather than strategies centered on interrupting normal activities to focus on the potential trauma (Galatzer-Levy, Burton, & Bonanno, 2012).

Expressive flexibility serves as another predictor of resilient outcomes (Bonanno, 2001; Consedine, Magai, & Bonanno, 2002; Gupta & Bonanno, 2011, Gross, 1999). Bonanno et al. (2004) first operationalized expressive flexibility as the capacity for enhancing and suppressing emotional facial expressions based on situational demands using a within-subjects paradigm. In a sample of New York City undergraduates who had entered college just prior to the 9/11 terrorist attacks, higher expressive flexibility (i.e., a greater ability to both up- and downregulate emotional expression) predicted lower psychological distress 2 years later. Follow-up studies that tracked this group of participants over extended periods of time provided convergent findings. One such study reported that expressive flexibility was similarly associated with a minimal-impact resilience trajectory of stable, low distress (Burton, Galatzer-Levy, & Bonanno, 2012). In another follow-up study, participants who demonstrated greater expressive flexibility in the presence of a subliminal threat prime evidenced better health and well-being as rated by their close friends (Westphal, Seivert, & Bonanno, 2010).

8.1.6.9 Genes

Research on the relationship between genetic variation and resilient outcomes in the presence of acute adversity is nascent. Presently, our lab is working on a new area of research examining single nucleotide polymorphisms in individuals who demonstrate the minimal-impact resilience trajectory following PTEs to determine whether genetic variation differentiates resilience from other response trajectories.

8.1.7 Conclusion

Even in the most challenging and aversive of circumstances, people carry on. Research on the human capacity for psychological resilience in the face of potential trauma and adversity has grown exponentially in the last decade. In order to guide future research and theory on psychological resilience, we present an integrative framework that conceptualizes the construct as a process comprising four temporal elements: baseline or pre-adversity adjustment, aversive circumstances, post-adversity resilient outcomes, and predictors of resilient outcomes. By highlighting both areas of existing knowledge and avenues worthy of further pursuit, our integrative temporal framework weaves together perspectives from multiple disciplines and sets the stage for the next phase of research on psychological resilience.

References

Ahern, J., Galea, S., Resnick, H., & Vlahov, D. (2004). Television images and probable posttraumatic stress disorder after September 11: The role of background characteristics, event exposures, and perievent panic. *Journal of Nervous and Mental Disease, 192*, 217–226.

Aldrich, D. P. (2012). *Building resilience: Social capital in post-disaster recovery*. Chicago, IL: University of Chicago Press.

Andersen, S. B., Karstoft, K.-I., Bertelsen, M., & Madsen, T. (2014). Latent trajectories of trauma symptoms and resilience: The 3-year longitudinal prospective USPER study of Danish veterans deployed in Afghanistan. *The Journal of Clinical Psychiatry, 75*(9), 1001–1008.

Aspinwall, L. G., & Taylor, S. E. (1997). A stitch in time: Self- regulation and proactive coping. *Psychological Bulletin, 121*, 417–436.

Berntsen, D., Johannessen, K. B., Thomsen, Y. D., Bertelsen, M., Hoyle, R. H., & Rubin, D. C. (2012). Peace and war: Trajectories of posttraumatic stress disorder symptoms before, during, and after military deployment in Afghanistan. *Psychological Science, 23*, 1557–1565. https://doi.org/10.1177/0956797612457389

Betancourt, T. S., & Khan, K. T. (2008). The mental health of children affected by armed conflict: Protective processes and pathways to resilience. *International Review of Psychiatry, 20*(3), 317–328. https://doi.org/10.1080/09540260802090363

Betancourt, T. S., McBain, R., Newnham, E. A., & Brennan, R. T. (2013). Trajectories of internalizing problems in war-affected sierra Leonean youth: Examining conflict and Postconflict factors. *Child Development, 84*(2), 455–470.

Bisconti, T. L., Bergeman, C. S., & Boker, S. M. (2004). Emotional well-being in recently bereaved widows: A dynamical systems approach. *Journals of Gerontology: Series B: Psychological Sciences & Social Sciences, 59B*(4), P158–P167.

Block, J. (1993). Studying personality the long way. In D. C. Funder, R. D. Parke, C. Tomlinson-Keasey, & K. Widaman (Eds.), *Studying lives through time: Personality and development* (pp. 9–41). Washington, DC: American Psychological Association.

Bloembergen, N., & Zewail, A. H. (1984). Energy redistribution in isolated molecules and the question of mode-selective laser chemistry revisited. New experiments on the dynamics of collisionless energy redistribution in molecules possibilities for laser-selective chemistry with subpicosecond pu. *The Journal of Physical Chemistry, 88*(23), 5459–5465. https://doi.org/10.1021/j150667a004

Bonanno, G. A., Papa, A., Lalande, K., Westphal, M., & Coifman, K. (2004). The importance of being flexible the ability to both enhance and suppress emotional expression predicts long-term adjustment. *Psychological Science, 15*, 482–487.

Bonanno, G. A., Brewin, C. R., Kaniasty, K., & La Greca, A. M. (2010). Weighing the costs of disaster: Consequences, risks, and resilience in individuals, families, and communities. *Psychological Science in the Public Interest, 11*, 1–49.

Boelen, P. A., de Keijser, J., van den Hout, M. A., & van den Bout, J. (2007). Treatment of complicated grief: A comparison between cognitive-behavioral therapy and supportive counseling. *Journal of Consulting and Clinical Psychology, 75*(2), 277–284.

Bombardier, C. H., Hoekstra, T., Dikmen, S., & Fann, J. R. (2016). Depression trajectories during the first year after traumatic brain injury. *Journal of Neurotrauma, 33*(23), 2115–2124.
Bonanno, G. A. (2001). Emotion self-regulation. [references]. In T. J. Mayne & G. A. Bonanno (Eds.), *Emotions: Current issues and future directions emotions and social behavior* (pp. 251–285). New York, NY: Guilford Press.
Bonanno, G. A. (2004). Loss, trauma, and human resilience: Have we underestimated the human capacity to thrive after extremely aversive events? *American Psychologist, 59*(1), 20–28.
Bonanno, G. A. (2005). Resilience in the face of loss and potential trauma. *Current Directions in Psychological Science, 14*(3), 135–138.
Bonanno, G. A., Brewin, C. R., Kaniasty, K., & La Greca, A. M. (2010). Weighing the costs of disaster: Consequences, risks, and resilience in individuals, families, and communities. *Psychological Science in the Public Interest, 11*(1), 1–49.
Bonanno, G. A., & Burton, C. L. (2013). Regulatory flexibility: An individual differences perspective on coping and emotion regulation. *Perspectives on Psychological Science, 8*(6), 591–612. https://doi.org/10.1177/1745691613504116
Bonanno, G. A., & Diminich, E. D. (2013). Annual research review: Positive adjustment to adversity–trajectories of minimal–impact resilience and emergent resilience. *Journal of Child Psychology and Psychiatry, 54*(4), 378–3401.
Bonanno, G. A., Field, N. P., Kovacevic, A., & Kaltman, S. (2002). Self-enhancement as a buffer against extreme adversity: Civil war in Bosnia and traumatic loss in the United States. *Personality and Social Psychology Bulletin, 28*(2), 184–196.
Bonanno, G. A., Galea, S., Bucciarelli, A., & Vlahov, D. (2006). Psychological resilience after disaster: New York City in the aftermath of the September 11th terrorist attack. *Psychological Science, 17*(3), 181–186. https://doi.org/10.1111/j.1467-9280.2006.01682.x
Bonanno, G. A., Galea, S., Bucciarelli, A., & Vlahov, D. (2007). What predicts psychological resilience after disaster? The role of demographics, resources, and life stress. *Journal of Consulting and Clinical Psychology, 75*(5), 671–682.
Bonanno, G. A., Ho, S. A. Y., Chan, J. C. K., Kwong, R. S. Y., Cheung, C. K. Y., Wong, C. P. Y., & Wong, V. C. W. (2008). Psychological resilience and dysfunction among hospitalized survivors of the SARS epidemic in Hong Kong: A latent class approach. *Health Psychology, 27*(5), 659–667. https://doi.org/10.1037/0278-6133.27.5.659
Bonanno, G. A., Keltner, D., Holen, A., & Horowitz, M. J. (1995). When avoiding unpleasant emotions might not be such a bad thing: Verbal-autonomic response dissociation and midlife conjugal bereavement. *Journal of Personality & Social Psychology, 69*(5), 975–989.
Bonanno, G. A., Kennedy, P., Galatzer-Levy, I. R., Lude, P., & Elfström, M. L. (2012). Trajectories of resilience, depression, and anxiety following spinal cord injury. *Rehabilitation Psychology, 57*(3), 236.
Bonanno, G. A., & Mancini, A. D. (2008). The human capacity to thrive in the face of potential trauma. *Pediatrics, 121*, 369–375.
Bonanno, G. A., Mancini, A. D., Horton, J. L., Powell, T. M., LeardMann, C. A., Boyko, E. J., … Smith, T. C. (2012). Trajectories of trauma symptoms and resilience in deployed US military service members: Prospective cohort study. *The British Journal of Psychiatry, 200*(4), 317–323. https://doi.org/10.1192/bjp.bp.111.096552
Bonanno, G. A., Neria, Y., Mancini, A., Coifman, K. G., Litz, B., & Insel, B. (2007). Is there more to complicated grief than depression and posttraumatic stress disorder? A test of incremental validity. *Journal of Abnormal Psychology, 116*(2), 342–351.
Bonanno, G. A., Papa, A., & O'Neill, K. (2001). Loss and human resilience. *Applied and Preventive Psychology, 10*, 193–206.
Bonanno, G. A., Rennicke, C., & Dekel, S. (2005). Self-enhancement among high-exposure survivors of the September 11th terrorist attack: Resilience or social maladjustment? *Journal of Personality and Social Psychology, 88*(6), 984–998.

Bonanno, G. A., Romero, S. A., & Klein, S. I. (2015). The temporal elements of psychological resilience: An integrative framework for the study of individuals, families, and communities. *Psychological Inquiry, 26*(2), 139–169.

Bonanno, G. A., Westphal, M., & Mancini, A. D. (2011). Resilience to loss and potential trauma. *Annual Review of Clinical Psychology., 7,* 511. https://doi.org/10.1146/annurev-clinpsy-032210-104526

Bonanno, G. A., Wortman, C. B., Lehman, D. R., Tweed, R. G., Haring, M., Sonnega, J., … Nesse, R. M. (2002). Resilience to loss and chronic grief: A prospective study from preloss to 18-months postloss. *Journal of Personality & Social Psychology, 83*(5), 1150–1164.

Bonanno, G. A. (2012). Uses and abuses of the resilience construct: Loss, trauma, and health-related adversities. *Social Science & Medicine, 74*, 753–756.

Breslau, N. (2001). Outcomes of posttraumatic stress disorder. *Journal of Clinical Psychiatry, 62*(Suppl 1), 55–59.

Breslau, N. (2009). The epidemiology of trauma, PTSD, and other posttrauma disorders. *Trauma, Violence, & Abuse, 10*(3), 198–210.

Breslau, N., Peterson, E. L., & Schultz, L. R. (2008). A second look at prior trauma and the post-traumatic stress disorder effects of subsequent trauma: A prospective epidemiological study. *Archives of General Psychiatry, 65*, 431–437.

Brewin, C. R., Andrews, B., & Valentine, J. D. (2000). Meta- analysis of risk factors for posttraumatic stress disorder in trauma-exposed adults. *Journal of Consulting and Clinical Psychology, 68*, 748–766.

Buckelew, S. P., Shutty, M. S., Jr., Hewett, J., Landon, T., Morrow, K., & Frank, R. G. (1990). Health locus of control, gender differences and adjustment to persistent pain. *Pain, 42*, 287–294.

Burton, C. L., Galatzer-Levy, I., & Bonanno, G. A. (2012). Expressive flexibility and long-term adjustment: A prospective study. Unpublished manuscript.

Burton, C. L., Galatzer-Levy, I. R., & Bonanno, G. A. (2015). Treatment type and demographic characteristics as predictors for cancer adjustment: Prospective trajectories of depressive symptoms in a population sample. *Health Psychology, 34*(6), 602.

Carr, V. J., Lewin, T. J., Webster, R. A., Kenardy, J. A., Hazell, P. L., & Carter, G. L. (1997). Psychosocial sequelae of the 1989 Newcastle earthquake: II. Exposure and morbidity profiles during the first 2 years post-disaster. *Psychological Medicine, 27*, 167–178.

Carver, C. S. (1998). Resilience and thriving: Issues, models, and linkages. *Journal of Social Issues, 54*(2), 245–266.

Cheng, C. (2001). Assessing coping flexibility in real-life and laboratory settings: A multimethod approach. *Journal of Personality and Social Psychology, 80*, 814–833.

Cicchetti, D., & Rogosch, F. A. (1997). The role of self-organization in the promotion of resilience in maltreated children. *Development and Psychopathology, 9*(04), 797–815.

Cicchetti, D., & Rogosch, F. A. (2009). Adaptive coping under conditions of extreme stress: Multilevel influences on the determinants of resilience in maltreated children. *New Directions for Child and Adolescent Development, 2009*(124), 47–59.

Cicchetti, D., & Rogosch, F. A. (2012). Gene by environment interaction and resilience: Effects of child maltreatment and serotonin, corticotropin releasing hormone, dopamine, and oxytocin genes. *Development and Psychopathology, 24*(2), 411.

Cicchetti, D., Rogosch, F. A., Lynch, M., & Holt, K. D. (1993). Resilience in maltreated children: Processes leading to adaptive outcome. *Development and Psychopathology, 5*(4), 629–647.

Conger, R. D., & Conger, K. J. (1992). A family process model of economic hardship and adjustment of early adolescent boys. *Child Development, 63*(3), 526.

Conger, R. D., & Conger, K. J. (2002). Resilience in Midwestern families: Selected findings from the first decade of a prospective, longitudinal study. *Journal of Marriage and Family, 64*(2), 361–373. https://doi.org/10.1111/j.1741-3737.2002.00361.x

Consedine, N. S., Magai, C., & Bonanno, G. A. (2002). Moder- ators of the emotion inhibition-health relationship: A review and research agenda. *Review of General Psychology, 6*, 204–228.

Copeland, W. E., Keeler, G., Angold, A., & Costello, E. J. (2007). Traumatic events and posttraumatic stress in childhood. *Archives of General Psychiatry, 64*(5), 577–584.

Currier, J. M., Neimeyer, R. A., & Berman, J. S. (2008). The effectiveness of psychotherapeutic interventions for bereaved persons: A comprehensive quantitative review. *Psychological Bulletin, 134*(5), 648–661.

Cutter, S. L., Barnes, L., Berry, M., Burton, C., Evans, E., Tate, E., & Webb, J. (2008). A place-based model for understanding community resilience to natural disasters. *Global Environmental Change, 18*(4), 598–606.

De Kloet, E. R., Derijk, R. H., & Meijer, O. C. (2011). Corticosteroid receptor involvement in the stress response. In *The handbook of stress* (pp. 47–75). Wiley-Blackwell.

DeRoon-Cassini, T. A., Mancini, A. D., Bonanno, G. A., & Rusch, M. D. (2010). Psychopathology and resilience following traumatic injury: A latent growth mixture model analysis. *Rehabilitation Psychology, 55*(1), 1–11. https://doi.org/10.1037/a0018601

Deshields, T., Tibbs, T., Fan, M. Y., & Taylor, M. (2006). Differences in patterns of depression after treatment for breast cancer. *Psycho-Oncology, 15*(5), 398–406.

DiRago, A., & Vaillant, G. (2007). Resilience in Inner City Youth: Childhood predictors of occupational status across the lifespan. *Journal of Youth and Adolescence, 36*(1), 61–70.

Donoho, C. J., Bonanno, G. A., Porter, B., Kearney, L., & Powell, T. M. (2017). A decade of war: Prospective trajectories of post-traumatic stress disorder symptoms among deployed US military personnel and the influence of combat exposure. *American Journal of Epidemiology, 186*(12), 1310–1318.

DuMont, K. A., Widom, C. S., & Czaja, S. J. (2007). Predictors of resilience in abused and neglected children grown-up: The role of individual and neighborhood characteristics. *Child Abuse & Neglect, 31*(3), 255–274.

Dumont, M., & Provost, M. A. (1999). Resilience in adolescents: Protective role of social support, coping strategies, self-esteem, and social activities on experience of stress and depression. *Journal of Youth and Adolescence, 28*(3), 343–363. https://doi.org/10.1023/A:1021637011732

Duncan, T. E., Duncan, S. C., & Strycker, L. A. (2006). An introduction to latent variable growth curve modeling: Concepts, issues, and applications. Quantitative methodology series (2nd ed., p. xii, 261 p.). Mahwah, NJ: Lawrence Erlbaum associates.

Egeland, B., Carlson, E., & Sroufe, L. A. (1993). Resilience as process. *Development and Psychopathology, 5*, 517.

Elder, G. H. (1998). The life course as developmental theory. *Child Development, 69*(1), 1–12. https://doi.org/10.1111/j.1467-8624.1998.tb06128.x

Elfström, M. L., Kennedy, P., Lude, P., & Taylor, N. (2007). Condition-related coping strategies in persons with spinal cord lesion: A cross-national validation of the spinal cord lesion-related coping strategies questionnaire in four community samples. *Spinal Cord, 45*(6), 420–428.

Fergus, S., & Zimmerman, M. A. (2004). Adolescent resilience: A framework for understanding healthy development in the face of risk. *Annual Review of Public Health, 26*, 399–419.

Ferguson, E., Matthews, G., & Cox, T. (1999). The appraisal of life events (ALE) scale: Reliability and validity. *British Journal of Health Psychology, 4*, 97–116.

Flores, E., Cicchetti, D., & Rogosch, F. A. (2005). Predictors of resilience in maltreated and non-maltreated Latino children. *Developmental Psychology, 41*(2), 338–351.

Foa, E. B., & Kozak, M. J. (1986). Emotional processing of fear: Exposure to corrective information. *Psychological Bulletin, 99*(1), 20–35. https://doi.org/10.1037/0033-2909.99.1.20

Foa, E. B., Rothbaum, B. O., Riggs, D. S., & Murdock, T. B. (1991). Treatment of posttraumatic stress disorder in rape victims: A comparison between cognitive-behavioral procedures and counseling. *Journal of Consulting and Clinical Psychology, 59*(5), 715–723. https://doi.org/10.1037/0022-006X.59.5.715

Frank, R. G., Umlauf, R. L., Wonderlich, S. A., Askanazi, G. S., Buckelew, S. P., & Elliott, T. R. (1987). Differences in coping styles among persons with spinal cord injury: A cluster- analytic approach. *Journal of Consulting and Clinical Psychology, 55*, 727–731.

Fredrickson, B. L., Tugade, M. M., Waugh, C. E., & Larkin, G. R. (2003). What good are positive emotions in crisis? A prospective study of resilience and emotions following the terrorist attacks on the United States on September 11th, 2001. *Journal of Personality and Social Psychology, 84*(2), 365.

Galatzer-Levy, I. R., & Bonanno, G. A. (2012). Beyond normality in the study of bereavement: Heterogeneity in depression outcomes following loss in older adults. *Social Science & Medicine, 74*(12), 1987–1994. https://doi.org/10.1016/j.socscimed.2012.02.022

Galatzer-Levy, I. R., & Bonanno, G. A. (2013). Heterogeneous patterns of stress over the four years of college: Associations with anxious attachment and Ego-resiliency. *Journal of Personality, 81*(5), 476–486. https://doi.org/10.1111/jopy.12010

Galatzer-Levy, I. R., & Bonanno, G. A. (2014). Optimism and death: Predicting the courses and consequences of depression trajectories in response to acute coronary syndrome.

Galatzer-Levy, I. R., Brown, A. D., Henn-Haase, C., Metzler, T. J., Neylan, T. C., & Marmar, C. R. (2013). Positive and negative emotion prospectively predict trajectories of resilience and distress among high-exposure police officers. *Emotion, 13*, 545. https://doi.org/10.1037/a0031314

Galatzer-Levy, I. R., & Bryant, R. A. (2013). 636,120 ways to have posttraumatic stress disorder. *Perspectives on Psychological Science, 8*(6), 651–662.

Galatzer-Levy, I. R., Burton, C. L., & Bonanno, G. A. (2012). Coping flexibility, potentially traumatic life events, and resilience: A prospective study of college student adjustment. *Journal of Social & Clinical Psychology, 31*, 542–567.

Galatzer-Levy, I. R., Huang, S. H., Bonanno, G. A. (2017). Trajectories of resilience and dysfunction following potential trauma: A meta-analytic review. Unpublished manuscript.

Galea, S., Ahern, J., Resnick, H., Kilpatrick, D., Bucuvalas, M., Gold, J., & Vlahov, D. (2002). Psychological sequelae of the September 11 terrorist attacks in New York City.[see comment]. *New England Journal of Medicine, 346*(13), 982–987.

Galea, S., Tracy, M., Norris, F., & Coffey, S. F. (2008). Financial and social circumstances and the incidence and course of PTSD in Mississippi during the first two years after hurricane Katrina. *Journal of Traumatic Stress, 21*, 357–368.

Galea, S., Brewin, C. R., Gruber, M., Jones, R. T., King, D. W., King, L. A., . . . Kessler, R. C. (2007). Exposure to hurricane- related stressors and mental illness after Hurricane Katrina. *Archives of General Psychiatry, 64*, 1427–1434.

Garmezy, N. (1972). Invulnerable children: The fact and fiction of competence and disadvantage. *American Journal of Orthopsychiatry, 42*, 328.

Galatzer-Levy, I. R., Madan, A., Neylan, T. C., Henn-Haase, C., & Marmar, C. R. (2011). Peritraumatic and trait dissociation differentiate police officers with resilient versus symptomatic trajectories of posttraumatic stress symptoms. *Journal of Traumatic Stress, 24*(5), 557–565.

Garmezy, N. (1993). Children in poverty: Resilience despite risk. *Psychiatry, 56*, 127–136.

Gralinski-Bakker, J. H., Hauser, S. T., Stott, C., Billings, R. L., & Allen, J. P. (2004). Markers of resilience and risk: Adult lives in a vulnerable population. *Research in Human Development, 1*(4), 291–326. https://doi.org/10.1207/s15427617rhd0104_4

Gross, J. J. (1999). Emotion regulation: Past, present, future. *Cognition & Emotion, 13*, 551–573.

Gupta, S., & Bonanno, G. A. (2010). Trait self-enhancement as a buffer against potentially traumatic events: A prospective study. *Psychological Trauma: Theory, Research, Practice, and Policy, 2*, 83–92.

Gupta, S., & Bonanno, G. A. (2011). Complicated grief and deficits in emotional expressive flexibility. *Journal of Abnormal Psychology, 120*, 635–643.

Hawley, D. R., & DeHaan, L. (1996). Toward a definition of family resilience: Integrating life-span and family perspectives. *Family Process, 35*(3), 283–298.

Helgeson, V. S., Snyder, P., & Seltman, H. (2004). Psychological and physical adjustment to breast Cancer over 4 years: Identifying distinct trajectories of change. *Health Psychology, 23*(1), 3–15. https://doi.org/10.1037/0278-6133.23.1.3

Hobfoll, S. E. (1989). Conservation of resources: A new attempt at conceptualizing stress. *American Psychologist, 44*(3), 513–524.

Hobfoll, S. E. (2002). Social and psychological resources and adaptation. *Review of General Psychology, 6*(4), 307–324.

Hobfoll, S. E., Canetti, D., Hall, B. J., Brom, D., Palmieri, P. A., Johnson, R. J., … Galea, S. (2011). Are community studies of psychological trauma's impact accurate? A study among Jews and Palestinians. *Psychological Assessment, 23*, 599–605.

Holling, C. S. (1973). Resilience and stability of ecological systems. *Annual Review of Ecology and Systematics, 4*, 1–23.

Hong, S.-B., Youssef, G. J., Song, S.-H., Choi, N.-H., Ryu, J., McDermott, B., … Kim, B.-N. (2014). Different clinical courses of children exposed to a single incident of psychological trauma: A 30-month prospective follow-up study. *Journal of Child Psychology and Psychiatry, 55*, 1226. https://doi.org/10.1111/jcpp.12241

Horowitz, M. J., Siegel, B., Holen, A., Bonanno, G. A., Milbrath, C., & Stinson, C. H. (1997). Diagnostic criteria for complicated grief disorder. *American Journal of Psychiatry, 154*(7), 904–910.

Hoven, C. W., Duarte, C. S., Lucas, C. P., Wu, P., Mandell, D. J., Goodwin, R. D., … Susser, E. (2005). Psychopathology among New York City public school children 6 months after September 11. *Archives of General Psychiatry, 62*, 545–552.

Huerta, F., & Horton, R. (1978). Coping behavior of elderly flood victims. *The Gerontologist, 18*(6), 541–546.

Johnson, H., & Thompson, A. (2008). The development and maintenance of post-traumatic stress disorder (PTSD) in civilian adult survivors of war trauma and torture: A review. *Clinical Psychology Review, 28*(1), 36–47. https://doi.org/10.1016/j.cpr.2007.01.017

Jones, E. (2006). Historical approaches to post-combat disorders. *Philosophical Transactions of the Royal Society B: Biological Sciences, 361*(1468), 533–542. https://doi.org/10.1098/rstb.2006.1814

Jones, E., Vermaas, R. H., McCartney, H., Beech, C., Palmer, I., Hyams, K., & Wessely, S. (2003). Flashbacks and post-traumatic stress disorder: The genesis of a 20th-century diagnosis. *The British Journal of Psychiatry, 182*(2), 158–163. https://doi.org/10.1192/bjp.02.231

Jones, E., & Wessely, S. (2005). *Shell shock to PTSD: Military psychiatry from 1900 to the Gulf war*. East Sussex, England: Psychology Press.

Kaniansty, K., & Norris, G. H. (2009). Distinctions that matter: Received social support, perceived social support, and social embeddedness after disasters. In Y. Neria, S. Galea, & F. N. Norris (Eds.), *Mental health and disasters* (pp. 175–200). New York: Cambridge University Press.

Kashdan, T. B., & Rottenberg, J. (2010). Psychological flexibility as a fundamental aspect of health. *Clinical Psychology Review, 30*, 865–878.

Kato, H., Asukai, N., Miyake, Y., Minakawa, K., & Nishiyama, A. (1996). Post-traumatic symptoms among younger and elderly evacuees in the early stages following the 1995 Hanshin-Awaji earthquake in Japan. *Acta Psychiatrica Scandinavica, 93*, 477–481.

Kawachi, I. (1999). Social capital and community effects on population and individual health. *Annals of the New York Academy of Sciences, 896*(1), 120–130.

Kennedy, P., Lude, P., Elfstrom, M. L., & Smithson, E. F. (2011). Psychological contributions to functional independence: A longitudinal investigation of spinal cord injury rehabilitation. *Archives of Physical Medicine and Rehabilitation, 92*, 597–602.

Kennedy, P., Marsh, N., Lowe, R., Grey, N., Short, E., & Rogers, B. (2000). A longitudinal analysis of psychological impact and coping strategies following spinal cord injury. *British Journal of Health Psychology, 5*, 157–172.

Knight, B. G., Gatz, M., Heller, K., & Bengtson, V. L. (2000). Age and emotional response to the Northridge earthquake: A longitudinal analysis. *Psychology and Aging, 15*, 627–634.

Krystal, J. H., & Neumeister, A. (2009). Noradrenergic and serotonergic mechanisms in the neurobiology of posttraumatic stress disorder and resilience. *Brain Research, 1293*, 13–23. https://doi.org/10.1016/j.brainres.2009.03.044.

La Greca, A. M., Lai, B. S., Llabre, M. M., Silverman, W. K., Vernberg, E. M., & Prinstein, M. J. (2013). Children's postdisaster trajectories of pts symptoms: Predicting chronic distress. In *Child & Youth Care Forum* (pp. 1–19). Berlin: Springer.

LaGreca, A., Silverman, W., Vernberg, E., & Prinstein, M. J. (1996). Symptoms of posttraumatic stress in children after Hurricane Andrew. A prospective study. *Journal of Consulting and Clinical Psychology, 64*, 712–723.

Lam, W. W. T., Bonanno, G. A., Mancini, A. D., Ho, S., Chan, M., Hung, W. K., … Fielding, R. (2010). Trajectories of psychological distress among Chinese women diagnosed with breast cancer. *Psycho-Oncology, 19*(10), 1044–1051. https://doi.org/10.1002/pon.1658

Lamprecht, F., & Sack, M. (2002). Posttraumatic stress disorder revisited. *Psychosomatic Medicine, 64*(2), 222–237.

Lazarus, R. S., & Folkman, S. (1984). *Stress, appraisal, and coping*. New York: Springer.

Le Brocque, R. M., Hendrikz, J., & Kenardy, J. A. (2010). The course of posttraumatic stress in children: Examination of recovery trajectories following traumatic injury. *Journal of Pediatric Psychology, 35*(6), 637–645. https://doi.org/10.1093/jpepsy/jsp050

Long, K., & Bonanno, G. A. (2017). Trait emotion predicts psychological distress following potentially traumatic events: A prospective study. Unpublished manuscript.

Lupien, S. J., McEwen, B. S., Gunnar, M. R., & Heim, C. (2009). Effects of stress throughout the lifespan on the brain, behaviour and cognition. *Nature Reviews Neuroscience, 10*(6), 434–445.

Luthar, S. S. (1999). *Poverty and children's adjustment*. Newbury Park, CA: Sage.

Luthar, S. S. (2003). *Resilience and vulnerability: Adaptation in the context of childhood adversities*. New York, NY: Cambridge University Press.

Luthar, S. S., Cicchetti, D., & Becker, B. (2000). The construct of resilience: A critical evaluation and guidelines for future work. *Child Development, 71*(3), 543–562.

Lyubomirsky, S., King, L. A., & Diener, E. (2005). The benefits of frequent positive affect. *Psychological Bulletin, 131*, 803–855.

Maccallum, F., Galatzer-Levy, I. R., & Bonanno, G. A. (2015). Trajectories of depression following spousal and child bereavement: A comparison of the heterogeneity in outcomes. *Journal of Psychiatric Research, 69*, 72–79.

Malgaroli, M., Galatzer-Levy, I. R., & Bonanno, G. A. (2017). Heterogeneity in trajectories of depression in response to divorce is associated with differential risk for mortality. *Clinical Psychological Science, 5*(5), 843–850.

Mancini, A. D., Bonanno, G. A., & Clark, A. E. (2011). Stepping off the hedonic treadmill: Latent class analyses of individual differences in response to major life events. *Journal of Individual Differences, 32*(3), 144–1582. https://doi.org/10.1027/1614-0001/a000047

Mancini, A. D., Littleton, H. L., & Grills, A. E. (2016). Can people benefit from acute stress? Social support, psychological improvement, and resilience after the Virginia Tech campus shootings. *Clinical Psychological Science, 4*(3), 401–417.

Masten, A. S. (2001). Ordinary magic: Resilience processes in development. *American Psychologist, 56*(3), 227–238.

Masten, A. S. (2007). Resilience in developing systems: Progress and promise as the fourth wave rises. *Development and Psychopathology, 19*(03), 921–930.

Masten, A. S., & Coatsworth, J. D. (1998). The development of competence in favorable and unfavorable environments: Lessons from research on successful children. *American Psychologist, 53*(2), 205–220. https://doi.org/10.1037/0003-066X.53.2.205

Masten, A. S., Hubbard, J. J., Gest, S. D., Tellegen, A., Garmezy, N., & Ramirez, M. (1999). Competence in the context of adversity: Pathways to resilience and maladaptation from childhood to late adolescence. *Development and Psychopathology, 11*(1), 143–169.

Masten, A. S., & Narayan, A. J. (2012). Child development in the context of disaster, war, and terrorism: Pathways of risk and resilience. *Annual Review of Psychology, 63*, 227–257.

McCrae, R. R., Costa, P. T., Ostendorf, F., Angleitner, A., Hrebick- ova, M., Avia, M. D., … Smith, P. B. (2000). Nature over nurture: Temperament, personality, and life span development. *Journal of Personality and Social Psychology, 78*, 173–186.

McCubbin, H. I., & McCubbin, M. A. (1988). Typologies of resilient families: Emerging roles of social class and ethnicity. *Family Relations, 37*(3), 247–254. https://doi.org/10.2307/584557

McNally, R. J. (2003). Progress and controversy in the study of posttraumatic stress disorder. *Annual Review of Psychology, 54*, 229–252.

McNally, R. J. (2012). The ontology of posttraumatic stress disorder: Natural kind, social construction, or causal system? *Clinical Psychology: Science and Practice, 19*(3), 220–228. https://doi.org/10.1111/cpsp.12001

Moskowitz, J. T., Folkman, S., & Acree, M. (2003). Do positive psychological states shed light on recovery from bereavement? Findings from a 3-year longitudinal study. *Death Studies, 27*, 471–500.

Muthén, B. (2004). Latent variable analysis: Growth mixture modeling and related techniques for longitudinal data. In D. Kaplan (Ed.), *Handbook of quantitative methodology for the social sciences* (pp. 345–368). Newbury Park, CA: Sage.

Nezu, A., & Carnevale, G. (1987). Interpersonal problem solving and coping reactions of Vietnam veterans with posttraumatic stress disorder. *Journal of Abnormal Psychology, 96*, 155–157.

Nugent, N. R., Tyrka, A. R., Carpenter, L. L., & Price, L. H. (2011). Gene–environment interactions: Early life stress and risk for depressive and anxiety disorders. *Psychopharmacology, 214*(1), 175–196.

Nolen-Hoeksema, S., & Morrow, J. (1991). A prospective study of depression and posttraumatic stress symptoms after a natural disaster: The 1989 Loma Prieta earthquake. *Journal of Personality and Social Psychology, 61*, 115–121.

Norris, F., Stevens, S., Pfefferbaum, B., Wyche, K., & Pfefferbaum, R. (2008). Community resilience as a metaphor, theory, set of capacities, and strategy for disaster readiness. *American Journal of Community Psychology, 41*(1–2), 127–150.

Norris, F. H. (1992). Epidemiology of trauma: Frequency and impact of different potentially traumatic events on different demographic groups. *Journal of Consulting and Clinical Psychology, 60*(3), 409.

Norris, F. H., Baker, C. K., Murphy, A. D., & Kaniasty, K. (2005). Social support mobilization and deterioration after Mexico's 1999 flood: Effects of context, gender, and time. *American Journal of Community Psychology, 36*(1–2), 15–28.

Norris, F. H., Friedman, M. J., Watson, P. J., Byrne, C. M., Diaz, E., & Kaniasty, K. (2002). 60,000 disaster victims speak: Part I. An empirical review of the empirical literature, 1981-2001. *Psychiatry, 65*(3), 207–239.

Norris, F. H., Tracy, M., & Galea, S. (2009). Looking for resilience: Understanding the longitudinal trajectories of responses to stress. *Social Science & Medicine, 68*, 2190–2198.

Offidani, E., & Ruini, C. (2012). Psychobiological correlates of allostatic overload in a healthy population. *Brain, Behavior, and Immunity, 26*(2), 284–291. https://doi.org/10.1016/j.bbi.2011.09.009

Ong, A. D., Bergeman, C. S., & Boker, S. M. (2009). Resilience comes of age: Defining features in later adulthood. *Journal of Personality, 77*(6), 1777–1804.

Ong, A. D., Bergeman, C. S., & Chow, S. M. (2010). Positive emotions as a basic building block of resilience in adulthood. In *Handbook of adult resilience* (pp. 81–93).

Ong, A. D., Fuller-Rowell, T. E., & Bonanno, G. A. (2010). Prospective predictors of positive emotions following spousal loss. *Psychology and Aging, 25*, 653–660.

Ong, A. D., Fuller-Rowell, T. E., Bonanno, G. A., & Almeida, D. M. (2011). Spousal loss predicts alterations in diurnal cortisol activity through prospective changes in positive emotion. *Health Psychology, 30*, 220–227.

Orcutt, H. K., Bonanno, G. A., Hannan, S. M., & Miron, L. R. (2014). Prospective trajectories of posttraumatic stress in college women following a campus mass shooting. *Journal of Traumatic Stress, 27*(3), 249–256. https://doi.org/10.1002/jts.21914

Okumura, T., Suzuki, K., Fukuda, A., Kohama, A., Takasu, N., Ishimatsu, S., & Hinohara, S. (1998). The Tokyo subway sarin attack: Disaster management, Part 1: Community emergency response. *Academic Emergency Medicine, 5*, 613–617.

Patterson, J. M. (1988). Families experiencing stress: I. The family adjustment and adaptation response model: II. Applying the FAAR model to health-related issues for intervention and research. *Family Systems Medicine, 6*(2), 202–237. https://doi.org/10.1037/h0089739

Patterson, J. M. (2002). Integrating family resilience and family stress theory. *Journal of Marriage and Family, 64*(2), 349–360. https://doi.org/10.2307/3600109

Pietrzak, R. H., Van Ness, P. H., Fried, T. R., Galea, S., & Norris, F. H. (2013). Trajectories of posttraumatic stress symptomatology in older persons affected by a large-magnitude disaster. *Journal of Psychiatric Research, 47*(4), 520–526.

Porter, B., Bonanno, G. A., Frasco, M., Dursa, E., Bossarte, R., & Boyko, E. (2017). Prospective post-traumatic stress disorder symptoms trajectories in active duty and separated military personnel. *Journal of Psychiatric Research, 89*, 55–64.

Prigerson, H. G., Horowitz, M. J., Jacobs, S. C., Parkes, C. M., Aslan, M., Goodkin, K., ... Maciejewski, P. K. (2009). Prolonged grief disorder: Psychometric validation of criteria proposed for DSM-V and ICD-11. *PLoS Medicine, 6*(8), e1000121. https://doi.org/10.1371/journal.pmed.1000121

Qouta, S., El-Sarraj, E., & Punamäki, R.-L. (2001). Mental flexibility as resiliency factor among children exposed to political violence. *International Journal of Psychology, 36*(1), 1–7. https://doi.org/10.1080/00207590042000010

Quale, A. J., & Schanke, A. K. (2010). Resilience in the face of coping with a severe physical injury: A study of trajectories of adjustment in a rehabilitation setting. *Rehabilitation Psychology, 55*, 12–22.

Reich, J. W., Zautra, A. J., & Hall, J. (2010). *Handbook of adult resilience: Concepts, methods, and applications*. New York, NY: Guilford.

Rutter, M. (1979). Protective factors in children's responses to stress and disadvantage. In M. W. Kent & J. E. Rolf (Eds.), *Primary prevention of psychopathology: Vol. 3: Social competence in children* (pp. 49–74). New Hampshire: University Press of New England.

Rutter, M. (1985). Resilience in the face of adversity: Protective factors and resistance to psychiatric disorder. *The British Journal of Psychiatry, 147*, 598–611. https://doi.org/10.1192/bjp.147.6.598

Rutter, M. (2002). The interplay of nature, nurture, and developmental influences: The challenge ahead for mental health. *Archives of General Psychiatry, 59*, 996–1000.

Ryff, C. D., & Singer, B. (2002). From social structure to biology: Integrative science in pursuit of human health and well-being. In S. J. Lopez & C. R. Snyder (Eds.), *Handbook of positive psychology* (pp. 541–555). Oxford: Oxford University Press.

Sampson, R. J., & Laub, J. H. (1992). Crime and deviance in the life course. *Annual Review of Sociology, 18*, 63–84. Retrieved from http://www.jstor.org/stable/2083446

Sampson, R. J., Raudenbush, S. W., & Earls, F. (1997). Neighborhoods and violent crime: A multilevel study of collective efficacy. *Science, 277*(5328), 918–924.

Sarapas, C., Cai, G., Bierer, L. M., Golier, J. A., Galea, S., Ising, M., ... Uhr, M. (2011). Genetic markers for PTSD risk and resilience among survivors of the World Trade Center attacks. *Disease Markers, 30*(2–3), 101–110.

Self-Brown, S., Lai, B. S., Thompson, J. E., McGill, T., & Kelley, M. L. (2013). Posttraumatic stress disorder symptom trajectories in hurricane Katrina affected youth. *Journal of Affective Disorders, 147*(1), 198–204.

Seligman, M. E., & Csikszentmihalyi, M. (2000). Special issue on happiness, excellence, and optimal human functioning. *American Psychologist, 55*(1), 5–183.

Shear, K., Frank, E., Houck, P. R., & Reynolds, C. F. (2005). Treatment of complicated grief: A randomized controlled trial. *Journal of the American Medical Association, 293*(21), 2601–2608.

Shepard, B. (2001). *A war of nerves: Soldiers and psychiatrists in the twentieth century*. Cambridge, MA: Harvard University Press.

Siegler, R. S. (1987). The perils of averaging data over strategies: An example from children's addition. *Journal of Experimental Psychology: General, 116*, 250. https://doi.org/10.1037/0096-3445.116.3.250

Smith, B., Dalen, J., Wiggins, K., Tooley, E., Christopher, P., & Bernard, J. (2008). The brief resilience scale: Assessing the ability to bounce back. *International Journal of Behavioral Medicine, 15*(3), 194–200. https://doi.org/10.1080/10705500802222972

Sonn, C. C., & Fisher, A. T. (1998). Sense of community: Community resilient responses to oppression and change. *Journal of Community Psychology, 26*(5), 457–472.

Sundin, J., Fear, N., Iversen, A., Rona, R., & Wessely, S. (2010). PTSD after deployment to Iraq: conflicting rates, conflicting claims. *Psychological Medicine, 40*(3), 367–382. https://doi.org/10.1017/S0033291709990791

Tang, C. S. (2007). Trajectory of traumatic stress symptoms in the aftermath of extreme natural disaster: A study of adult Thai survivors of the 2004 southeast Asian earthquake and tsunami. *The Journal of Nervous and Mental Disease, 195*(1), 54–59.

Ullman, J., & Newcomb, M. (1999). I felt the earth move: A prospective study of the 1994 Northridge earthquake. In L. Cohen, P. Slomkowski, & C. Robins (Eds.), *Historical and geographical influences on psychopathology* (p. 2170246). Mahwah, NJ: Lawrence Erlbaum Associates.

Vaillant, G. E., & Davis, J. T. (2000). Social/emotional intelligence and midlife resilience in schoolboys with low tested intelligence. *American Journal of Orthopsychiatry, 70*(2), 215–222. https://doi.org/10.1037/h0087783

Vasterman, P., Yzermans, C. J., & Dirkzwager, A. J. E. (2005). The role of the media and media hypes in the aftermath of disasters. *Epidemiologic Reviews, 27*(1), 107–114.

Vernberg, E. M., La Greca, A. M., Silverman, W. K., & Prinstein, M. J. (1996). Prediction of posttraumatic stress symptoms in children after hurricane Andrew. *Journal of Abnormal Psychology, 105*, 237–248.

Walsh, F. (1996). The concept of family resilience: Crisis and challenge. *Family Process, 35*(3), 261–281. https://doi.org/10.1111/j.1545-5300.1996.00261.x

Walsh, F. (2006). *Strengthening family resilience* (2nd ed). New York, NY: Guilford Press.

Walsh, F. (2013). Community-based practice applications of a family resilience framework. In D. S. Becvar (Ed.), *Handbook of family resilience* (pp. 65–82). New York: Springer.

Waters, E., & Sroufe, L. A. (1983). Social competence as a developmental construct. *Developmental Review, 3*(1), 79–97. https://doi.org/10.1016/0273-2297(83)90010-2

Weems, C. F., Pina, A. A., Costa, N. M., Watts, S. E., Taylor, L. K., & Cannon, M. F. (2007). Predisaster trait anxiety and nega- tive affect predict posttraumatic stress in youths after hurricane Katrina. *Journal of Consulting and Clinical Psychology, 75*, 154–159.

Weems, C. F., Taylor, L. K., Cannon, M. F., Marino, R. C., Romano, D. M., Scott, B. G., … Triplett, V. (2010). Post traumatic stress, context, and the lingering effects of the hurricane Katrina disaster among ethnic minority youth. *Journal of Abnormal Child Psychology, 38*, 49–56.

Werner, E. E. (1985). Stress and protective factors in childrens lives. In A. R. Nicol (Ed.), *Longitudinal studies in child psychology and psychiatry* (pp. 335–355). New York: Wiley.

Werner, E. E. (1993). Risk, resilience, and recovery: Perspectives from the Kauai longitudinal study. *Development and Psychopathology, 5*(4), 503–515.

Werner, E. E. (1995). Resilience in development. *Current Directions in Psychological Science, 4*(3), 81–85.

Werner, E. E., Bierman, J. M., & French, F. E. (1971). *The children of Kauai: A longitudinal study from the prenatal period to age ten*. Honolulu: University of Hawaii Press.

Werner, E. E., & Smith, R. S. (1982). *Vulnerable but invincible: A longitudinal study of resilient children and youth*. New York: McGraw Hill.

Werner, E. E., & Smith, R. S. (1977). *Kauai's children come of age*. Honolulu: University Press of Hawaii.

Werner, E. E., & Smith, R. S. (1992). *Overcoming the odds: High risk children from birth to adulthood*. Ithaca, NY: Cornell University Press.

Westphal, M., Seivert, N. H., & Bonanno, G. A. (2010). Expressive flexibility. *Emotion, 10*, 92–100.

Wyman, P. A., Cowen, E. L., Work, W. C., Raoof, A., Gribble, P. A., Parker, G. R., & Wannon, M. (1992). Interviews with children who experienced major life stress: Family and child attributes that predict resilient outcomes. *Journal of the American Academy of Child & Adolescent Psychiatry, 31*(5), 904–910.

Yehuda, R., & Flory, J. D. (2007). Differentiating biological correlates of risk, PTSD, and resilience following trauma exposure. *Journal of Traumatic Stress, 20*(4), 435–447. https://doi.org/10.1002/jts.20260

Zhu, Z., Galatzer-Levy, I. R., & Bonanno, G. A. (2014). Heterogeneous depression responses to chronic pain onset among middle-aged adults: A prospective study. *Psychiatry Research, 217*(1), 60–66.

Chapter 9
Conclusions and Panel Discussion

Jennie G. Noll and Idan Shalev

The chapters included in this volume represent the bulk of the proceedings from "New Frontiers in the Biology of Stress, Maltreatment and Trauma: Opportunities for translation, resilience and reversibility," held from September 30 to October 1, 2015. Li and Danese focus on Biological Embedding of Child Maltreatment through Inflammation. This chapter provides an overview of the role of inflammation as a key mediator in explaining the link between childhood adversity and risk of psychopathology, with a specific focus on the effects of childhood maltreatment on depression. The authors conclude with the possibility of targeting the inflammatory system in depressed individuals with a history of childhood adversity by using anti-inflammatory drugs.

Heim discusses the Psychobiological Consequences of Child Maltreatment. This chapter describes results implicating the nervous, immune, glucocorticoid, and oxytocin systems, as well as physical changes in the brain as key mediators and/or outcomes of early life adversity. The role of genetics and epigenetics in moderating and mediating these processes, respectively, is also discussed. The author concludes with a call for mechanism-informed interventions for survivors of child abuse by targeting specific biomarkers and physiological systems and by employing longitudinal prospective designs.

Ellis's chapter, Toward an Adaptation-Based Approach to Resilience, provides a novel perspective on resiliency in the face of early adversity. Ellis presents an adaptation-based approach, incorporating a developmental programming framework, to better understand and explain why some individuals thrive while others struggle

J. G. Noll (✉)
The Pennsylvania State University, USA
e-mail: jgn3@psu.edu

I. Shalev
Department of Biobehavioral Health, The Pennsylvania State University,
State College, PA, USA

© Springer International Publishing AG, part of Springer Nature 2018

J. G. Noll, I. Shalev (eds.), *The Biology of Early Life Stress*, Child Maltreatment Solutions Network, https://doi.org/10.1007/978-3-319-72589-5_9

when exposed to harsh environments. This perspective offers a different approach by defining the stress-induced changes as "specialization," that is, a developmental adaptation that enhances the survival of individuals in an ecologically relevant environment. Ellis further discusses the tradeoffs that are inherent in this approach and offers a new look for designing and thinking about education, policy, and intervention studies for children who grow up in harsh environments.

Rock, Geier, Noll, and De Bellis address the role of Brain Development in Maltreated Children With and Without PTSD. This chapter summarizes key neurobiological findings in maltreated children, focusing on developmental effects, sex differences, cognitive skills, and the development of post-traumatic stress disorder (PTSD) among affected children. The authors highlight the advantageous perspective of considering the effects of maltreatment when treating survivors of childhood trauma as well as considering individual differences in devising new treatment strategies.

Herringa discusses the topic of Childhood Maltreatment and Pediatric PTSD: Abnormalities in threat neural circuitry. This chapter elaborates on the effects of childhood maltreatment and PTSD, with an emphasis on functional brain abnormalities such as threat processing. Herringa proposes an adaptive model wherein childhood maltreatment leads to heightened reactivity in the amygdala, which helps to fine-tune threat processing, and thus enables the child to survive in harsh conditions. The author further discusses other brain regulatory systems related to maladaptive outcomes among survivors of child maltreatment and how delineating neurobiological mechanisms can advance prevention and intervention studies.

Altamirano, Basile, and Carrion present the topic of Pediatric Posttraumatic Stress, incorporating behavioral, emotional, anatomical, and biological aspects. This chapter further elucidates treatment options for survivors, highlighting individual therapies as well as large-scale preventive interventions such as yoga and mindfulness curricula at schools. The authors' aim is to implement evidence-based research for pediatric PTSD treatment that could inform policy changes.

Bouvette-Turcot, Meaney, and O'Donnell discuss Epigenetics and Early Life Adversity: Current Evidence and Considerations for Epigenetic Studies in the Context of Child Maltreatment. This chapter considers the importance of epigenetic processes in the context of early life adversity. The authors describe the mechanisms by which epigenetics can leave a fingerprint that can result in an enduring phenotype of dysfunctional physiological and neurobiological function. Both pre-clinical and clinical studies are discussed, along with important methodological considerations. The authors conclude that further in-depth research is needed to advance our understanding of epigenetic processes before they can be implemented in clinical studies.

Long and Bonano describe An Integrative Temporal Framework for Psychological Resilience. This concluding chapter extends upon previous models of resiliency and provides a new conceptual framework. The authors highlight four temporally related elements, how they unfold over time, and their essential roles in adaptive functioning in the face of trauma. The authors further provide predictors of emergent resilience, including caregiver–child relationships, cognitive skills and emotions, flexibility, and genes. The framework presented in the chapter sets the stage for further research on resilience for survivors of early trauma.

The final session of the conference included an open discussion in which audience members were encouraged to ask questions of the distinguished panel. The focus of the panel discussion was not to glean clarification of the research presented—there was ample time to do that at the end of each talk—but rather to ask the panel about the next essential steps in the progression of this science and to provide advice for the next generation of scientists in this area. The group was charged with identifying the essential "stepping stones" to rapid progression of ideas and collaborative efforts that had not yet been fully realized until this unique group was brought together. Most of those who presented their work at the conference have produced chapters for this volume. However, several individuals were unable to contribute a chapter (Appendix A includes the conference agenda). The discussion excerpted herewith includes both presenters who contributed chapters and those who did not. Out of respect for each scholar, the names of those who responded to questions are not published in this panel discussion. Instead, the tenor and each question and its answer are summarized so as to protect the identity of those who asked questions as well as those who responded. In cases in which several individuals responded to questions, P1, P2, P3,...PX correspond to sequential responses in the order delivered and do not necessarily denote differing individuals. It should also be noted that the following questions and answers were edited to be succinct summaries of transcripts and represent the basic points that were conveyed in the panel discussion. These summaries are the interpretations of the authors of this chapter and are not meant to reflect word-for-word quotations of speakers.

Question 1: Are there community-based interventions that are designed to mitigate the impact of stress on child development?

Answer. P1: There is work funded by the Institute for Educational Sciences addressing achievement disparities in this country, especially for highly mobile children where it might be very difficult to intervene with a strategy that requires 12 months or 2 years of intervention. The most important thing for families in a shelter environment is to stabilize their environment in good quality housing with good quality care available for their children. In collaboration with shelters over time, we can create early childhood programs that are very accessible for these highly mobile families—something that other programs like Head Start cannot accommodate. What is needed is a practical program that can be implemented in a short period of time, such as Tools of the Mind (Bodrova & Leong, 2007). Tools of the Mind is an intervention for child development with a particular focus on executive function skills delivered in short-term boosts to facilitate "top-down" control skills. The intervention has been developed with several strategies in mind. One strategy is to include the intervention in classrooms for 3–5-year-olds to provide children a "boost" before they enter regular preschool or kindergarten programs. The approach trains teachers to tweak regular classroom activities to enhance the reflection training and practice of cognitive flexibility. There is also a family component to basically educate parents about little things they can do every day to help their children practice some of these self-control skills. Also, the connection between stress and sleep regulation is becoming increasingly important to understand within the context of these types of interventions. Hence, it will be exciting to be able to measure change in the biological processes that have been discussed at this conference.

Question 2: Can you say a bit more about regulatory flexibility being adaptive?

Answer. P1: Flexibility is adaptive not because one can do multiple things, but because one can do different things. You might develop a propensity toward a certain strategy because you're good at it or because you're adapting to your environment. But the question is, "Can you *not* use that strategy in another situation?" For example, if you grow up in a hostile environment and then are removed from that environment, can you readapt? Feedback is another piece of flexibility. If you get the feedback that something is not working, can you switch, or are you too rigid? We need to be able to measure people's behavior in situations—not simply self-report measures—because you get a lot more complexity.

P2: Even if our interventions are designed to promote adaptation in one context, how do we know that those skills won't be maladaptive in another context? For example, for very disadvantaged children, we want them to succeed in a regular school context where a completely different set of skills is required than what is required in chaotic home or neighborhood environments. Naturally occurring adaptation, perhaps being as comfortable on the street as in the school environment, requires a lot of flexibility because not everything we might want a kid to do in a middle-class school environment is going to work out for them on dangerous streets.

P3: Then there is the notion of "early inoculation," or experience with mild stressors preparing one for being able to adapt. Some of the primate work suggests that certain types of preparations for upcoming stressors, like early experience with separation when it's going to be permanent later on, can help the young primate deal with that eventual loss. But timing seems to be crucial. The same experience that can have long-term inoculating effects may actually have long-term adverse consequences if introduced at the wrong developmental point. Do we know anything more about the rules that govern these types of inoculation, and how would we come to better understand those processes? What about overprotecting children?

Kids need practice in dealing with things on their own. For example, they need to learn how to fall safely if they're learning to ice skate. Experiencing separations like having babysitters or going off to daycare will help prepare a child to go off to school. There's also a whole different literature on preparing children for anticipated stressors: e.g., at what age can you really prepare a child for the separations of hospitalization, or medical treatments, and that sort of thing? You know, there are some things you can do cognitively, but children need to have some practice. But from every study I've ever looked at, the response to stressors looks very nonlinear. It looks like some challenges, some stressors, are positive, but then you move rapidly into a counterproductive phase. I assume it's developmentally very sensitive, just the way we know that it is in primates with separation and as we know it is with things like developing protection from asthma. It matters when you're exposed to microorganisms: if you're exposed late, the same microorganisms can trigger really bad reactions; if you're exposed early, it can develop a stronger immune system.

Question 3: Coming from an animal and genetics background do you think that maybe we're measuring children too far apart, that measurement is not necessarily getting at these processes for adolescents who are at risk or are in family systems where you can't necessarily get the history through the par-

ents? What do you think can be done to help better capture these dynamic processes?

Answer. P1: Examining data right after an event, and at very proximal time points, you may still be able to model the same parameters as more rapid and even longer term effects. We did, for example, a spinal cord injury study, and to ascertain what happens right after the injury, we see fairly recognizable patterns. But we need to remember, since everything we measure has error, if you get finer, and finer, and finer, you're just getting more error, which will need to be modeled. It may be best to have very proximal data and go from there.

P2: Our measurement timeframes need to fit with the processes and change that we're trying to capture. There are some things that, if you measure it too quickly, you can't get a sense of the directionality because everything is embedded in covariation. If you take too long, you miss all the in-between processes and cascades. The situation, for example, of people living in an emergency shelter provides a very unique opportunity to look very closely at some of the processes of change—day-to-day or even moment-to-moment—providing some important opportunities to watch and understand adaptation as it's unfolding.

P3: Depending on what the topic is, there are also modal points that are very important to capture. For example, when researching how people react to getting cancer, there are clear points of change, and we have to know what those points are and get data around those particular points. And so depending on what the topic is, whether it's life in a shelter or a traumatic incident, there typically modal points that are theoretically (or developmentally) important to describe in addition to those most proximal to the event.

Question 4: While it seems that flexibility is certainly important, do you also agree that stability is important, or the ability to predict or have an expectation about the future? For example, there is some work showing that plasticity might be extremely useful in limited developmental periods but detrimental if constant.

Answer. P1: You can think about curvilinear relationships: being so flexible that you change at a whim. Context sensitivity, for example, assumes that one is reading the context accurately, figuring out what is needed, and then adjusting to that need.

P2: This may be just another general reflection on flexibility. One of the most powerful ways that parents regulate the lives of kids is to read the environment and then adjust; parents adjust their behavior in many ways, even to impending danger, for example. If you take a warm, permissive parent and move that parent into a dangerous environment like the inner city of Chicago, that parent will shift strategies to protect the well-being of her children. She will become extremely strict, for example, while maintaining the warmth that provides access and emotional stability.

Question 5: How can the findings presented here be shared? How do we engage the community, both survivors and those who are advocating for survivors?

Answer. P1: Special dissemination events can be organized, perhaps by the funding agencies that could involve politicians, advocacy groups, and even victims. If these key stakeholders could be allocated time to speak about how the research informed public health policies and clinical care, this could allow conversations about how we could bring common research together with the expectations of advocacy groups.

P2: An often-quoted line is that you are not really a scientist unless you can communicate your findings to the public (Babbie, 2007). But that's really become more of an uphill battle because of the immensity of the media.

P3: There is a real concern, on the part of very good neuroscientists, about how neuroscience is being perceived in much of the public discourse as giving simple, deterministic answers to complicated issues. There is a "dumbing down" and having conceptions (or misconceptions) maintained because journalists wanted sound bites. We need to get out of that habit. There is no readily available answer except to better educate those who are conducting the interviews and making sure that science is being given its due without dumbing it down.

P3: The question is really, "To whom are you communicating?" If you're communicating to politicians, for example, they may be driven by ideology and are not interested in the evidence base. We need to strive to educate politicians about evidence-based decision-making, perhaps bringing in the economics of the argument. If you're disseminating for the sake of communication, then you want to be understood. If you're disseminating for the sake of change, then you need to know who are the best agents of change and how do you work with them in partnership. Patient groups often turn out to be the best agent of change.

P4: If we can appeal based on health care cost and other public costs, that will also be helpful in imploring change.

P5: You need a really great and compelling story that grabs people. And you have to wrap it in stories, not just data, graphs, and slides, as these things just go into the vapor. You have to grab people at the level of emotions on the stories, and you have to have a compelling message. So, as a field, we need to really work with marketing and advertising people to deliver a potentially profound message.

P6: This is an extremely important issue and question and is one of the most compelling reasons a resilience framework makes sense. Although it's inherently a risk and resilience framework, communicating the goals of the work, recruiting participants, and communicating the message is very different when it's within the framework of trying to understand how adversity affects the lives of children and what we can do about it to promote healthier outcomes.

We also need to learn *how* to communicate—to get trained in how to communicate and to practice doing so. We need to practice getting the message right and understanding the goal of your talk and who the audience is. We need to get over the assumption that we should not talk to the press because "they always get it wrong" or they "misquote." What we need is formal training on how to package our ideas and talk to the media. We also underestimate how much our data can speak if we package them in compelling ways. For example, things may look hopeless if you just present averages, but when you show the individual variation, that lots of kids are actually doing well, and there are ways to improve kids' well-being, this is what is compelling. The people in this room (and at this conference) need to be communicating with each other, because otherwise it will all be filtered through ambassadors who may not represent the best of our science. We don't want others to speak for us. It is vitally important that we take on that task of communicating with our participants, our legislatures, and the press.

Question 6: What is the next essential step in this science; in the translation—particularly at glucocorticoid receptor or the molecular level—to the level of the person or the child, to the family or the community?

P1: It will be extremely important that we have multiple levels of consideration requiring multidisciplinary teams. We need venues for collaboration, like this conference, to understand how these things work independently and together. One of the most important next steps will be to mobilize the funders and funding to do the kind of research that has been presented here.

P2: Many of us face methodological or analytical issues when trying to collect longitudinal data representing multiple levels of analysis, everything from the genomic level up to societal levels or community levels and everything in between. While we are pretty good at analyzing data within a single level of analysis, we're not very good at crossing levels. We don't know the rules, for example, of how to model the relationship between changes in glucocorticoid expression, cortisol output, and emotional reactivity in a sensible way over time. In many cases, you're collecting the data on different time scales, representing differing degrees of precision. The whole issue of causality gets muddled even if you have longitudinal data because there are external events that can cause changes in gene methylation or expression, which in turn feeds back up to biological processes. So the question of, "what causes what" in the traditional way won't work. We need a new set of rules, a new set of guidelines, and some standards by which we can understand relationships between events or measures between one level of analysis and another. And then how do we test the efficacy of those models?

P3: We live on a planet where political conflict and climate change have forced people to come together to understand what happens in these crises and to think ahead about preparing for disaster. It has been illuminating to watch these processes when people from very different levels of analysis try to figure out what should be done. We have lots of issues facing us that require more integrated approaches across levels. Some of the folks at other levels or other fields like ecology have some interesting statistical modeling strategies for the behavior of dynamic systems that are complex. There have been some gains in these fields that perhaps we can learn from.

P4: Many scientists in this area are torn between two different directions. One is that we look at the sense of exposure period for risk. For example in some of our analyses, 14 years of age seems to be a very critical spot in that both males and females who experience maltreatment at that age have the most predictive response for showing or developing major depression later on in life. But this comes from pooling cross-sectional research together. An obvious choice is to conduct the definitive longitudinal study to target specific periods of risk and malleability—neurobiologically, molecularly, and clinically. The other is the strong emphasis on the distinction between psychiatric conditions with and without maltreatment, which we call the "ecophenotype." We need to be more persuasive in this argument, and we need additional data that would allow us to parse out psychiatric diagnosis from maltreatment, and vice versa.

P5: Wouldn't it be great to turn to pediatricians and say, "Here's a test that you can use at the level of the individual child to see whether the adversity that you know has occurred has had an impact that is predictive of a particular outcome," and have it be deliverable and usable within their clinical practice? And then to deal with the issues of comorbidities in pediatric settings? These comorbidities probably have a common origin but are interfacing.

P6: And we get asked all the time, "How can we find an objective diagnostic test to verify experiences?" In order to be definitive, we need to do a better job to establish causality because most of the research in this area is cross-sectional, especially when we study adults and long-term consequences. We may need to combine large-scale longitudinal cohorts because we cannot start at zero and go until 80 years. We may need to capitalize on what we have already established to answer new questions.

Reversibility is also very important. Many of the biological systems that we think are changed by early adversity could be modified or counteracted. We should not be afraid to also explore novel pharmacological ways to reach the consequences of child maltreatment. For example, one of the talks in this conference showed that FK506 Binding Protein 5 (FKBP5) is one target that could be modified or blocked to normalize glucocorticoid regulation. Animal models can also be informed by human research findings to answer such questions and help in establishing causality.

P7: We should also be thinking about how to work with practitioners to more fully understand *how* interventions work. If we understand how they work, we might be able to then understand how we can modify them to make them work better for more people.

P8: We should all be moving toward understanding the casual mechanisms associated with the impact of maltreatment of children. A recent article in *Nature* showcased why interdisciplinary research matters and how funding agencies don't really understand because they are supportive of only one discipline. We really need to combine forces, combine different expertise, to see advancements that will come from new technologies.

P9: In another sense, multidisciplinary doesn't necessarily mean multilevel per se. In other words, "How does the field of child maltreatment grow with the field of stress, with the field of aging, with the field of obesity?" How do different fields grow together, to inform each other's science?

Question 7: What is the best intervention that's never been tested?

Answer. P1: Rough play, as a kind of inoculation. I'm sort of piggybacking on Tremblay's (Paquette, Carbonneau, Dubeau, Bigras, & Tremblay, 2003) work, but interactive highly social vigorous physical play.

P3: Like reintroducing recess. Get kids playing more.

P4: We should develop a study to understand how children from high-adversity contexts become good at learning, memory, reasoning, problems solving, etc. Then use this information to leverage better interventions.

P5: There is some good evidence beginning to emerge that things like play and exercise could be very valuable and have an impact on plasticity.

Question 8: What is your advice or charge to the next generation of scientists?

Answer. P1: Be ready to train kids from the very beginning to be interested in interdisciplinary research.

P2: Study individual differences.

P3: Embrace the new technologies. Be very proficient in the area of big data and big data analytics.

P4: Break down silos. Perhaps to begin the breakdown is to get rid of the concept of stress altogether. We should be talking about adversities, individual differences, and reversibility.

P5: Don't be afraid to think outside of the box. The only way we can make real progress is to not repeat what has been done before. Be creative. And be integrative, talk to people, and go to conferences like this one.

Appendix A: New Frontiers in the Biology of Stress, Maltreatment, and Trauma: Opportunities for Translation, Resilience, and Reversibility

Conference Agenda

Day 1: Wednesday, September 30	
8:30–8:35 a.m.	Call to Order
8:35–8:55 a.m.	Introductory Remarks
	Network Director Jennie Noll, Ph.D., Penn State.
	President Eric Barron, Ph.D., Penn State
Session I	**Endocrinology and Immunology**
	Integrative speaker: Christine Heim, Ph.D.
	Moderator: Idan Shalev, Ph.D., Penn State
9:00–9:35 a.m.	Andrea Danese, M.D., Ph.D., King's College London
9:35–10:10 a.m.	Hannah Schreier, Ph.D., Penn State
10:10–10:45 a.m.	Bruce Ellis, Ph.D., University of Arizona
10:45–11:00 a.m.	*Coffee Break*
11:00–11:45 a.m.	Christine Heim, Ph.D., Penn State and Charité Universitätsmedizin Berlin
11:45 a.m.–Noon	Open Discussion
Noon–1:00 p.m.	*Lunch*
Session II	**Brain Development**
	Integrative speaker: Martin Teicher, M.D., Ph.D.
	Moderator: Carlo Panlilio, Ph.D., Penn State
1:00–1:35 p.m.	Michael De Bellis, M.D., Ph.D., Duke University
1:35–2:10 p.m.	Ryan Herringa, M.D., Ph.D., University of Wisconsin
2:10–2:45 p.m.	Victor Carrión, M.D., Stanford University
2:45–3:30 p.m.	Martin Teicher, M.D., Ph.D., McLean Hospital and Harvard Medical School
3:30–3:45 p.m.	Open Discussion

(continued)

Day 2: Thursday, October 1	
8:30–8:35 a.m.	Introductory Remarks
	Network Director Jennie Noll, Ph.D., Penn State.
Session III	**Genomics**
	Integrative speaker: Michael Meaney, Ph.D.
	Moderator: Chad Shenk, Ph.D., Penn State
8:35–9:10 a.m.	Kieran O'Donnell, Ph.D., McGill University
9:10–9:45 a.m.	Bekh Bradley-Davino, Ph.D., Emory University and Atlanta VAMC
9:45–10:20 a.m.	Idan Shalev, Ph.D., Penn State
10:20–10:30 a.m.	*Coffee Break*
10:30–11:15 a.m.	Michael Meaney, Ph.D., McGill University
11:15–11:30 a.m.	Open Discussion
11:30–12:30 p.m.	*Lunch*
Session IV	**Resilience and Reversibility**
	Moderator: Jennie Noll, Ph.D., Penn State
12:30–1:15 p.m.	Ann Masten, Ph.D., University of Minnesota
1:15–2:00 p.m.	George Bonanno, Ph.D., Columbia University
2:00–2:45 p.m.	Stephen Suomi, Ph.D., NICHD
2:45–3:00 p.m.	Questions and Open Discussion
Session V	**Opportunities for Translation Panel Discussion**
	Moderator: Jennie Noll, Ph.D., Penn State
3:00–3:45 p.m.	Integrative Speakers, plus session attendees, will convene in front of the conference audience to field questions, facilitate conversation, and enhance discussion
3:45–3:50 p.m.	Closing Remarks (Jennie Noll, Ph.D.)

References

Babbie, E. R. (2007). Writing social research. In *The practice of social research* (p. 508). Belmont, CA: Thompson Wadsworth.

Bodrova, E., & Leong, D. (2007). *Tools of the mind: The Vygotskian approach to early childhood education* (2nd ed.). Columbus, OH: Merrill.

Paquette, D., Carbonneau, R., Dubeau, D., Bigras, M., & Tremblay, R. (2003). Prevalence of father-child rough-and-tumble play and physical aggression in preschool children. *European Journal of Psychology of Education, 18*(2), 171–189. Retrieved from http://www.jstor.org/stable/23420447

Index

© Springer International Publishing AG, part of Springer Nature 2018

J. G. Noll, I. Shalev (eds.), *The Biology of Early Life Stress*, Child Maltreatment Solutions Network, https://doi.org/10.1007/978-3-319-72589-5

The manufacturer's authorised representative in the EU is Springer Nature Customer Service Centre GmbH, Europaplatz 3, 69115 Heidelberg, Germany. If you have any concerns regarding our products, please contact ProductSafety@springernature.com

Printed and bound by CPI Group (UK) Ltd, Croydon, CR0 4YY
30/09/2026
02225658-0018